PRESERVING LIFE

PRESERVING LIFE

Public Policy and the Life
Not Worth Living

Richard Sherlock

LOYOLA UNIVERSITY PRESS

Chicago

Loyola University Press
3441 North Ashland Avenue
Chicago, Illinois 60657

Library of Congress Cataloging in Publication Data
Sherlock, Richard.
Preserving life.
Bibliography: p. 302
Includes index.
1. Right to die—Law and legislation.   2. Medical
ethics.   I. Title.
K3611.E95S45   1986   344'.0419   86-21347
ISBN 0-8294-0526-7   342.4419

Design by C. L. Tornatore

For Peggy, Thomas and Alexandra

And where if not in God should lie the criterion for the ultimate value of a life? In the subjective will to live? On this rating many a genius is excelled by half-wits. In the judgement of society? If so, it would soon be found that opinion as to which lives were socially valuable or valueless would be determined by the requirements of the moment and therefore by arbitrary decisions; one group of human beings after another would in this way be condemned to extermination. The distinction between life that is worth living and life that is not worth living must sooner or later destroy itself.

Dietrich Bonhoeffer
Ethics

Acknowledgments

Over the years that this book has been in preparation, I have incurred many debts to others, most of them too numerous to mention. A few, however, must be named here. Discussions with Roger Barrus, Gary Atkinson, Dave Mall, Bob Barry, O.P., John McDermott, S.J., James Bopp, Lynn Wardle, Cliff Perry, and Dave Thomasma helped to clarify my argument and its limits. Bill Bartholome, M.D. gave encouragement at many stages of my work and taught me more about pediatric medicine than I ever thought I could learn. Likewise, John Mullooly, M.D. has been a source of encouragement and enlightenment. Arthur Dyck has been a teacher and friend for many years and his encouragement was crucial at an early stage in the clarification of my ideas. Numerous physicians at the University of Tennessee College of Medicine helped to increase my knowledge of their art, as did colleagues in the Faculty of Medicine at McGill University in Montreal.

The first version of this manuscript was completed when I was a member of the Theology Department at Fordham University. The intellectual stimulation of that environment was extremely useful in forcing the clarification of my ideas and their defense. The final work on this manuscript was done while I was a Senior Research Scholar at the Center for Bioethics of the Clinical Research Institute of Montreal. The Center and the Institute are superior places for work in bioethics. The Director of the Center, Dr. David Roy, and my fellow researcher, John Williams, were always very helpful and supportive of my work; I shall always cherish my time spent there. At the Center Ms. Chantal Grenier expertly typed the manuscript from what must have seemed like incomprehensible notes on an early draft. Fr. Robert Clark, S.J., my editor at Loyola University Press, labored strenuously to make this book more readable and coherent, for which I am very grateful. All these friends and institutions made this book better than it might have been, but none are responsible for what remains.

Contents

Contents

Introduction

Three Difficult Cases

1. Baby Jane Doe—the Right to Treatment

On October 11, 1983 at St. Charles Hospital in Port Jefferson, New York, a baby girl, known only as "Jane Doe," was born with myelomeningocele, commonly known as spina bifida, and supposedly hydrocephalus—water on the brain—and microcephaly—an abnormally small head or brain. The facts of this case are disputed and their interpretation even more so; therefore, one must proceed with caution in any description. St. Charles Hospital is a medium-sized community facility which, though excellent, is not equipped to offer the best, state-of-the-art care in complicated cases such as that of Baby Doe. As soon as possible that day, Baby Doe was transferred to the hospital affiliated with the Medical School of the State University of New York at Stony Brook, which could provide the treatment needed by Baby Doe.[1]

The parents of Baby Doe consented to the transfer of their daughter on the advice of physicians both at St. Charles and at Stony Brook. They knew that the transfer was for surgery nec-

1

essary to prolong the life of their daughter. The trial record clearly shows that the need for surgery was stated to the parents and that they verbally consented to it. But they did not sign a consent form. At Stony Brook the parents later consulted further with medical specialists, counselors, and priests from their church; they decided they would not permit surgery on their daughter. It seems clear from the record that the parents believed that Baby Jane would die very quickly—in twenty-four to forty-eight hours—and that this belief played a role in their decision to withhold treatment.[2]

From a purely medical standpoint, Baby Jane's need for surgery cannot be seriously doubted. Spina bifida involves a lesion in the spinal cord and an open sac of loose tissue and fluid at the point of lesion. Unless surgery is performed to drain the sac and close the lesion, the opening would be the site of repeated major infections which most certainly would cause the death of Baby Doe before age two, if not sooner. She could die at any time; indeed, she may very well be dead before this is published.[3]

Press reports that her life span would be twenty years with surgery stem from a quite erroneous interpretation of trial testimony. One of the physicians treating Baby Jane was asked about her life span. He answered: "there is really no way of placing a limit on it if surgery is performed." Then he was asked, "could it conceivably be twenty years?" He answered, "Yes." But neither he nor any other expert ever stated that twenty years was the limit of her life span.

Surgery to close the lesion in her spine would do nothing, however, to alter either the physical or mental handicaps with which she would be faced if she were allowed to live as long as possible by those who must care for her. Inevitably, these facts and their interpretation by her parents and physicians became central in deciding about her care. It is here, however, that the supposed facts become less clear and their interpretation much more debatable. The location of the lesion was in the sacral area of the spine, a location associated with the fewest long-term handicaps for the infant.[4] Just what these handicaps would be was a matter of prognosis, guesswork, and dispute. One ex-

2

pert, Dr. George Newman, a pediatric neurologist at Stony Brook whose advice was taken very seriously by Baby Jane's parents, testified in court that she would be bedridden; but his written prognosis, made when he first examined her, concluded that she would be able to walk with braces.[5] He also testified that her arms were spastic; but the chairman of his own department testified at the same time that the arms had normal movement and muscle tone.[6] It was also likely that the lesion would cause her to lose bladder and bowel control; surgical repair would not restore them.

The most important and most disputed of the supposed facts concerned the condition of her brain and the prognosis for her mental development. At various times it was reported that she had a small head, hydrocephalus—usually associated with a large head, or microcephaly. The first of these appears to be false: her head size was normal in proportion to her body. The other two are true. Hydrocephalus refers to water or fluid on the brain and is compatible with microcephaly, in which the brain mass is not fully developed and fluid fills the remainder of the intracranial cavity.[7]

But what count are the inferences one may draw from these facts regarding the future life of Baby Jane; here there is an enormous range of opinion. Dr. Newman painted a quite bleak picture: "It is very unlikely that she is going to develop any cognitive skills whatsoever."[8] His department chairman, Dr. Alan Butler, the pediatric neurosurgeon who would have done the surgery, was more optimistic. He claimed that "we have reasonably to expect that this child might be able to sit up, look around, be aware of parents and friends."[9] An outside expert on the treatment of spina bifida, Dr. David McLone of Children's Hospital in Chicago, disagreed further. He concluded from what was available in the public record that "normal development" was possible.[10]

If there is a consensus of professional opinion, it is only that Dr. McLone may be too optimistic; but beyond that, the disagreement between Dr. Newman and Dr. Butler is fundamental. If Dr. Newman's guess is correct, many reasonable people would conclude that a decision not to perform surgery was within the bounds of reasonable morality. But if Dr. Butler is correct, I submit that many of us would conclude that, however much her life may differ from ours, the simple pleasures of Baby Jane's life could make it worthwhile and meaningful for her and that surgery to preserve it should be performed.

The parents, however, took Dr. Newman's advice and refused surgery. They deliberately chose a shorter life for their daughter as opposed to the longer one described by Dr. Newman.

A few days after their decision, an anonymous tip on the case was given to A. Lawrence Washburn, a lawyer whose home is in Vermont but whose municipal-bond practice is heavily involved in New York. Washburn is widely known for his crusading activities on behalf of the pro-life movement. He immediately petitioned the courts of New York on behalf of the infant whom, he claimed, was being medically neglected and deprived of necessary medical care. Washburn, of course, had no connection with the case until this point, had no relation to the baby, had very little knowledge of her condition and was, in fact, ignorant of the medical record of the care given to Baby Jane. To remedy this deficiency the court appointed another lawyer, again unknown to the case, to act as a guardian *ad litem* for Baby Jane. As such he was empowered to review the relevant record, to question the parents, physicians, and other staff persons, and to recommend to the court whether it should declare the child neglected and order surgery. The guardian *ad litem* concluded that surgery was in the best interests of the child. The trial judge agreed and ordered surgery.[11]

Before surgery could actually be performed, the parents and the physicians appealed the decision. Over the course of the next month, their decision to refuse surgery was upheld by the state's intermediate court of appeal and by the highest court in the state. At both levels, however, the courts sidestepped the questions over which these parents and the guardian *ad litem* agonized. At the first appellate level, the essential finding was that Baby Jane was not neglected, since her parents had followed the recommendations of licensed physicians. Since physicians disagree on these matters, it was permissible for the parents to accept the professional advice of one over another, provided the advice were offered by a licensed physician with appropriate training. If they were properly informed and not coerced into their choice, it should be respected. No attempt was made to challenge the medical recommendation itself, to see if it actually reflected the best interests of Baby Jane.[12]

The decision of the state's highest court was even further removed from the questions that generated the controversy. It held that state law did not permit the intervention of Washburn in the first place and that, as a result, the course of the legal proceedings since then had been invalid. The concern of the court was that the law has traditionally been very suspicious of third-party intervention in the complex and delicate lives of families. To balance the families' need for autonomy with the necessity of protecting children from abuse and neglect, special agencies of government have been established with the power to intervene and seek from the courts protection of the children's best interests. But only in such agencies, they concluded, has that power been lodged; it would create an ominous precedent to hold that third parties with no connection to a family, either professional or genealogical, can intervene in matters as sensitive as this whenever they believe the family has acted incorrectly. Furthermore, the court agreed with the appeals court that, since the parents had followed the advice of licensed physicians, they could not be charged with neglect.[13]

One would have thought that this decision would have ended the discussions about the care of Baby Jane, except in academic journals and forums. Such hope was optimistic. After the state courts had disposed of the case, the federal government began its involvement, to determine if Baby Jane was being discriminated against in ways that violated federal law. The government's claim was that section 504 of the Rehabilitation Act of 1973 prohibited institutions that received federal funds from discriminating against persons who are physically or mentally handicapped.[14] Since federal medicare and medicaid funds were a major resource of Stony Brook Hospital, the government claimed that it had the power to investigate the case and make its own determination about whether this child was being deprived of medical care solely because of her supposed physical and mental disabilities. If so, the theory ran, the government could withhold further funds from Stony Brook Hospital, a clearly coercive move that almost certainly would have compelled the hospital to make every effort to operate.

But the government needed access to the hospital records to determine if discrimination were taking place. They needed to know precisely what the condition of the baby was originally. Where was the lesion? How large was it? How much of the brain was present and what portion, cerebellum, midbrain, brainstem, and so forth? Only the complete hospital record could answer these questions. At this point the hospital refused to release the record and the government filed suit in federal court to obtain it.

Though it dismissed some of the contentions the hospital made in its defense, the federal district court rejected the central contentions of the government: 1) that it had jurisdiction in the case, and 2) that if discrimination occurred, the hospital was at fault. On the latter claim the court held that the hospital is powerless to operate with neither the consent of the parents nor a court order secured under state neglect statutes. Since it had neither, and since it remained willing to operate once consent was secured, it could not be held to have discriminated against Baby Jane. The government's contention that failure to seek authorization under the state neglect laws for the surgery constituted discrimination would, the court reasoned, be an unreasonable expansion of the duties of the hospital.[15]

The crucial matter, however, was whether the government had any authority to intervene here. On this point both the federal district and appelate courts ruled against the government. They both held that, given the language and legislative history of section 504, it would be unreasonable to conclude that Congress intended it to cover such cases. Hence the government had no power to compel the hospital to permit an examination of the record or to perform the surgery.[16]

At this point the government has appealed this ruling to the Supreme Court, where it is uncertain what the ultimate fate of this legal wrangling will be. Nor do we know how long Baby

Jane will live or with how much discomfort and pain. Nonetheless, it seems certain that Baby Jane will be remembered long after she passes from mortality. However anonymous, her name has indelibly marked our public consciousness. For in her case we see in microcosm the complex and exceedingly controversial decisions that are now forced on us as individuals and as a polity. As we grope for answers to these controversies, Baby Jane will not be forgotten.

2. *Ellen Bouvia—the Right to Die*

At the same time that Baby Jane journeys toward death without the medical care that might have prevented it, another woman three thousand miles away raises her own voice for the right to end through starvation her life, one filled with more suffering than Baby Jane will ever know.

Ellen Bouvia is a twenty-six-year-old woman who is completely paralyzed from cerebral palsy. She has partial use of one hand, sufficient to operate an electric wheelchair, and she can eat solid food if fed by someone else. Other than that she requires the assistance of others for even the most routine and private functions. In the preceding years she had obtained a college degree, been married, and tried to live alone with the assistance of friends and a personal care aide. But in the last year her husband left her, she dropped out of school, and she returned to live with her family. Ultimately, she concluded that, for her, life as a total invalid, always being cared for by others, was not worth the effort. She obtained admission to the psychiatric ward of a California hospital by claiming that she was suicidal, whereupon she refused to take any nourishment. In short, she proposed to starve herself to death.[17]

But she chose to do so in a setting that was established to preserve life, not to aid people in ending their lives. Hence a conflict of moral vision and will was inevitable. The hospital sought to force-feed Ms. Bouvia and she sued in court for the right to proceed as she wished. Her attorney persuaded her to take nourishment while her case went to court, but after that she wanted to be dead rather than live in the manner in which she would be forced to live. Once her competency had been established by professional assessment, the claim she advanced was stark: a competent adult ought to have the right to do what he or she wishes to do with his or her life, even if that means ending it. The analogy was to the right of the patient to refuse any medical care one does not want, even care that may be necessary to save life, such as dialysis. We do not force dialysis on patients. Why then should we force-feed Ellen Bouvia?[18]

This analogy is not exact, however, and the hospital challenged her on it. The person who does not want dialysis may refuse to come in for treatment. The hospital has no power to send agents out to bring people in for treatment against their will. But Ms. Bouvia did not simply wish to refuse medical care available at the hospital; she asked the hospital to keep her while she died. Given the requirements of institutional hygiene, that would have inevitably meant that the hospital and its staff would have to provide a considerable amount of personal care to Ms. Bouvia while they waited and watched her die in their hands. This, they concluded, they could not do, especially in an institution whose mission was the saving of life.

At this writing a lower court has sided with the hospital and permitted the force feeding by tube of Ms. Bouvia.[19] She has appealed and the appeal awaits its turn in the legal system.

Like Baby Jane, Ellen Bouvia has left a permanent mark on our public consciousness, whatever the outcome of her legal maneuverings and appeals. How should the public values upheld by the hospital and its staff relate to the private and disparate choices of persons like Ellen Bouvia, who find action consistent with the public values is intolerable for them? Should the hospital be required to compromise its adherence to the public ethic of the goodness of life and the duty to care for it, by acceding to Ms. Bouvia's demands? If so, what of other matters of conscience where hospitals and physicians may be pitted against patients' values, such as abortion? If a complete dismissal of the moral tenor of the hospital is an unacceptable result, what is the alternative for Ms. Bouvia? Should she be sent home, where she will be faced with the inevitably more demanding, but perhaps less successful, ministrations of her family? Should she be sent somewhere else? Where? To an apartment with a live-in aide to provide the necessary hygienic care? Even if this were possible, could we expect the aide to sit passively at her side while she slowly starves to death? Or should Ellen Bouvia die alone in the stench of her excrement which she cannot dispose of herself? Would it not rather be more merciful to kill her outright, to give her to drink of Socrates' hemlock which we now forbid her?

Both Baby Jane and Ellen Bouvia raise enormously troubling issues for a people and a society dedicated to the values of life and liberty. Neither of these unfortunate human beings is in that well-known and well-talked about—but ill-defined—category of "terminally ill." They both would live substantial lengths of time except for the deliberate decisions that they or others make about their care. Nor are they isolated cases except in the irrelevant sense that every case is different, with its own texture and its own factual nuances. As the capacities of modern medicine to sustain life increase, so too do the queries: at what cost? with what consequences for the quality of individual lives, for the stability and coherence of our moral convictions and for the preservation of the public values lying at the core of our civilization? Thirty years ago Baby Jane would have been dead by now, either from the failure of less advanced and sophisticated surgical techniques or from repeated infections that would have rapidly overwhelmed the limited antibiotic armamentarium available then. Even in the case of Ellen Bouvia, our capacity to reduce the complications of cerebral palsy and to institute feeding with a nasogastric tube now make possible the very intervention permitted by the court and desired by the hospital.

If these cases and countless others remind us of the questions that medicine now forces upon us, they do so in ways that inevitably transcend the limits of private moral choice. To be sure, Baby Jane's parents and physicians have choices to make, based on the facts as they perceive them and the beliefs they hold. So do Ellen Bouvia and the people she has asked to care for her in her own way. Although the agents of these choices may be private, the import of the choices is public. A society such as ours that is committed to the right to life and hence value of each human being, that is heir to centuries of common law development of such a right, cannot be indifferent when parents and physicians deliberately choose a course of action they know will drastically shorten the life of a handicapped infant. Nor can we avoid the public choices that Ms. Bouvia forces on us. She cannot take her life in private; she needs the assistance of public institutions and agents in whose moral tenor and actions we all have a stake. To note only the most obvious point here, our polity surely must prevent the lethal medical neglect that some parents, however sincere, inflict on their children.

3. A Cancer Patient—The Right to Refuse Treatment

This stake has been developed in a century of medical neglect law and has been upheld in a controversial case just at the time that Baby Jane was deprived of surgery. In this Tennessee case an adolescent girl had Ewing's sarcoma that had relapsed from an earlier remission.[20] Without aggressive treatment death was certain. With it, the child might have her life saved, in the ambiguous language of the oncologist where five years of disease free survival is defined as cure. Yet the fact that this child had relapsed into her disease made any positive prognosis very uncertain. At most it could be claimed that she had about a 30–40 per cent chance of having her life saved even with the most aggressive therapy available.[21]

She and her family understood these facts, but they profoundly disagreed with the conclusion to which such facts seemed to point. They asserted a faith in God and his healing powers and a corresponding right to ignore the advice of physicians and to seek instead a healing miracle that they believed their God would offer. In attempting to exercise this right, they ran directly into the beliefs of the physicians that the girl need-

10

ed standard medical therapy and their willingness to press their case in court. Unlike the courts of New York, the courts in Tennessee relied on a century of precedent and found that parents may not choose death over life for a minor, irrespective of the religious sincerity of the claims made by the family of the child.[22] Whatever the law may permit these adults to do because of their faith, it cannot permit them to demand the same measure of obedience from those too young to choose. Unfortunately, the court viewed the case in quite stark life-or-death terms and ignored nuances that seemed to blur such an analysis. Had the court taken seriously the uncertainties in this case, its resolution may not have been as easily developed along the lines of established precedent.

The court's position rested on its view of the necessity of treatment to save the life of the child. In such situations the common law is clear and the court faithfully applied it. However, when the life of the child is not at stake or when experimental procedures are proposed, the courts are traditionally less willing to second guess parents by ordering medical care that they have refused. At the very least, the precedent in these cases is less certain and more flexible than those where a choice between life and death for the child is more certain.[23] But if this case were in fact as uncertain in its potential for cure as it appears to have been, should not the response of the court be more nuanced and flexible? Perhaps, but the point remains that this court adopted a century-old tradition of medical-neglect law that, applied in the manner of this court, leads to conclusions radically different from those reached in the case of Baby Jane.

When, then, does failure to provide therapy become neglect or providing it transgress the plausible limits of the best interest of the individual human being? These questions cannot be strictly private matters of personal and familial choice. As the courts both in New York and Tennessee implicitly recognized, these must be matters of public choice, however much we are at a loss for certainty in our answers or perfect clarity in our decision making in such cases. We wish these cases would go away but they will not: they remain to challenge us, even after we have formulated what we believe to be the best public responses.

Issues of Biomedical Ethics and Principles
for Public Policy

These observations form the horizon within which this book examines the most pressing questions of biomedical ethics and public policy. I will, of course, examine the teachings of moralists and physicians who want to provide a morally correct resolution of these issues of life and death. Given the importance attached to these inquiries, one could hardly avoid a serious dialogue with them. But my aims are somewhat different. This examination will proceed in light of principles and convictions that underpin our life together in community, that define the essence of our polity, and that establish the limits of acceptable public practices. To reach this point we will need to understand the essential core of liberal regimes as well as the relations between political regimes and public policies. In the context of such an inquiry, we can explore the central questions of life and death in modern medicine as issues requiring public choice and can sketch the minimum terms of an acceptable public resolution of these same issues. In essence we will demonstrate the nature of what must be an acceptable public resolution of these matters, one enshrined in law, institutional guidelines, and committee decisions, as well as the limits of such a resolution insofar as a morally perfect solution to these sorts of cases is concerned.

If policy appears only in the context of a specific political community, so too must it envision actual practice as well. Policy ill-suited to its object is readily ignored; sporadic attempts to enforce it only increase the sense of injustice. But we shall see in the final chapter that, in practice, a public policy giving voice to a deep sense of the equal worth of all human beings and deliberately eschewing claims about a "poor quality of life" will not impinge unjustly on clinical practice nor lead to inhumane forms of care. In fact, for all the rhetoric about quality-of-life judgments in medicine, in actual practice their role in decision making is less obvious and their necessary place in clinical choice is far from certain. Except for certain classes of infants, much of what appears under this banner can equally well be described in other terms, terms that do not raise the sorts of issues that will concern us here.

One of the enduring functions of law and public policy is to call attention to the central convictions of communal life against the momentary passions that at some point engulf us all. "Law," wrote Roscoe Pound, "prevents the sacrifice of ultimate interests, individual and social, to the more pressing but less weighty immediate interests."[24] In this sense, law closes off options even as it articulates the essence of our public commitments. This function of law is at best a minimalist function. Such rules can exclude that which simply cannot be permitted but they cannot in any sense dictate where justice actually will be found in any specific case. It excludes the utterly unacceptable and points us in the direction in which an acceptable solution is most likely to be found but it cannot tell us before hand what that solution is to be. To ask more of law, to ask it to regulate all the minutiae of human experience, is to pervert law itself and distort our search for justice, even the minimal justice of which we imperfect people are capable.

This will appear as an imperfect solution to the adherents of the viewpoints that now seem to dominate the discussion of such questions. Those who assert that law and policy can completely regulate individual activity and choice will find my view of the relation of policy to practice less deductive and more complex than tidy resolutions of every case would require. To those who believe in the myth of the open society, closing off any horizon of choice will appear as an unacceptable limitation. That these may be imperfections I readily admit. But they are imperfections that are coeval with human existence, for which none of the political, moral, or jurisprudential theorists of any age has found a solution.

In what follows we begin by developing the nature of regimes as entities bound together by a common vision of the good and the just. In chapter two the central conviction of liberal regimes regarding the equal worth of each human life is argued for, partly by showing how that conviction emerges from and is given voice by the central founding theorists of the liberal tradition. From this basis we proceed to examine four fundamental issues of public choice which are currently much disputed: care for defective newborns *versus* infanticide, care for gravely or terminally ill adults *versus* euthanasia, suicide, and abortion. In the final chapter we take up the matter of actual clinical practice and the relation of policy to practice noted above.

CHAPTER ONE

Political Regimes and Public Policies

Classical Foundations

Socratic Quest and Platonic Vision

In books eight and nine of Plato's *Politeria*, or *Republic*, Socrates turns his attention from the regime in speech that he has just founded for his interlocuters, Glaucon and Adeimantus, to the various alternatives that present themselves in actual political practice. Socrates does not, of course, confuse this inquiry with what has gone before, just as Plato does not confuse the regime founded by Socrates with that founded by the Athenian Stranger in the *Laws*. While Socrates' maneuver in books eight and nine seems simple enough, however, it is actually a profound inquiry into the most significant of political things. Here Socrates seeks to illumine, dialectically, the political good itself by examining the various forms in which it partially presents itself. As such, his discussion moves at several levels of speech and action. At the most superficial level, Socrates offers a description of the fundamental alternatives of political organization, such as democracy, oligarchy, and so forth. In this sense, he offers us a political science of various forms of government, similar to modern descriptive analyses.[1] This description, however, is transcended even as it is presented, by Socrates' parallel description of the type of citizen and the way of life characteristic of these different regimes. In a way the "form of government" description is only an entrée to the examination of the differing habits, passions, and ruling opinions that flourish in and define the existence of various regimes. These opinions about the right and the good and the passions and habits they engender are the essence of political regimes; only insofar as a person permits one's soul to be ruled by such opinions and passions can one permit one's body to be ruled by a regime that embodies these same ruling opinions.[2]

In none of these cases does Socrates suppose that he is describing perfect justice. Insofar as it is possible, he has already founded the just regime in speech, or so it appears. Socrates' act of founding is, however, impossible apart from a wisdom that belies his claim to be only a midwife. Now, in order for his interlocuters to see even a modest portion of justice he must show them how it will differ from the political alternatives that are displayed in books eight and nine. Thus the unity of justice and wisdom that is at the heart of the teaching of the *Republic* is brought to its deepest point precisely where Socrates displays his knowledge of the fundamental alternative regimes and the phenomena that are coeval with them.

Socrates' examination of these differing regimes points to the distinction between justice itself and the political forms in which it is embedded, as well as to a connection between political regimes and the qualities of character that each regime fosters. These insights are, in fact, inseparable. In practice, political justice is found in specific regimes, not regimes in speech. It thus encounters men and women of widely varying temperaments and opinions, characteristics that are nurtured in the soil of various regimes. Political justice must take these characteristics into account, and govern in light of them. In other words, it appears that justice itself must be differentiated; it must appear as many and not one. But, if Socrates' teaching in the *Republic* is

16

taken seriously justice is one. It is regimes that differ. Thus the tension appears between justice itself and that which presents itself as justice in the various regimes in which it inevitably appears.[3]

In this respect Socrates does not spend much time in offering criticisms of these lesser regimes. Their deficiencies are obvious, especially in light of the teaching in the dialogue as a whole. But the deficiencies that distinguish these regimes are not themselves grounds for calling their legitimacy or their own species of justice into question. Only in the worst case, tyranny, must we engage in the total criticism of a political order that is so common in recent times. This criticism is, of course, necessitated by Socrates' desire to wean Glaucon from his attraction to the tyrannic life. But the lack of such a total assault on other regimes, imperfect though they surely are, does point us in a fundamental direction.

Even if Plato would have accepted as worthwhile a study of ethics in the independent manner that Aristotle's account seems to suppose, such a treatment could not reveal the politically just or proper. On this point Aristotle would agree. Unlike many moderns, for whom a moral critique of political forms and practices is an endless exercise, Plato teaches the distinction between politics and morality. Socrates, of course, constantly pursued a philosophic investigation and thereby criticism of political practices. But the Socratic examination of political life illumines precisely the distinction between the requirements of political justice and public practice and those that might govern the moral agent himself in special and unique cases. For the purely moral examination of human activity seeks to uncover the just and the right in the circumstances of individual choice and then, insofar as possible, to systematize these reflections as universal guides for human activity in all possible similar cases. In this manner the study of ethics begins with a species, human being, who is faced with a moral choice from which the moralist determines the right and the good in such a case and then formulates a general rule for all such cases.[4]

Political practice and public policy, however, cannot begin

17

with the species man as such. Rather, actual political rule begins with individual human beings, each an imperfect copy of the species, each with his or her own capacities, habits, and passions. Furthermore, in practice ordinary political rule cannot take account of the extraordinary and the unusual. This point is at the very center of Plato's teaching about the most extraordinary person of Socrates.[5] Rather politics must treat in the first instance, the usual and the regular. It must abstract from the unusual and the extraordinary and govern in light of the expected and the probable. Hence, politics emerges as a fundamentally distinct enterprise from the abstract formulations and contextual exception clauses found in all branches of morality. Political justice entails an abstraction from the pursuit of justice per se, which must be concerned with the ambiguities of context and the good for human beings *per se*. This teaching, lying near the center of classical, premodern political thought, one can observe in every major political philosopher of the Western tradition from Plato to St. Thomas.[6] Since political justice must concern itself with differences among regimes and the characteristics of their citizens, it cannot determine in the abstract, apart from these differences, where the best alternatives will be found in public decision making nor will citizens be likely to act in the manner required by that alternative and having committed themselves in another direction it may be unjust for such citizens to depart. The success of any such departures would therefore be unlikely and their adoption imprudent and perhaps unjust.

These observations are especially telling for the case of complex problems that involve matters of central significance to the regime. Precisely in these cases morality seems to require the nuanced flexibility which political practice and law cannot provide to the requisite degree. In the matters that concern us here this point is amply demonstrated. In any polity, especially a liberal regime, it cannot be a matter of indifference whether a person lives or dies by the hand of another. Nor, if the fetus is granted human standing, can abortion be regarded as the strictly private matter it has come to be seen as in our day. If our polity must stand for life in these instances, it must do so in

18

ways that will inevitably entail bypassing the nuances of extraordinary cases. What is necessary as a rule for the vast majority of cases may not provide the flexibility of complete justice in some unique and special instances.

In this regard written law is conspicuously absent from the just regime founded by Socrates. It is only in this regime, however, and nowhere else in the Platonic corpus, that the notion of selective infanticide of defective newborn infants is endorsed. In Plato's only other treatment of the issue, the written law of the *Laws* is different.[7] The public policy of actual regimes, embodied as it must be in written law, simply cannot distinguish in an adequate manner those cases where death is preferable to life from those cases where killing must be prohibited as murder. Just as in the cases of mercy killing, euthanasia, or any number of other core issues that will concern us later in this book political practice seems to presume the value of each life and abstracts from the extraordinary cases in which justice appears in a different form, no matter how compelling that form may appear to be.

In the same manner, liberal societies cannot sanction slavery in any instance, irrespective of whether or not it might be true that some blacks would have preferred to remain under the secure aegis of their masters. The political justice of liberal regimes necessarily presumes that liberty in this sense is a core good and only those lacking in reason or blinded by their experiences would wish to remain enslaved.

In saying this I hold no brief for the proposition that slavery could ever be justified in any situation. What I am calling attention to is the way in which liberal regimes expel slavery from their midst, not on grounds of abstract morality but because it cannot be squared with the fundamental conception of justice under which such a regime governs its citizens and establishes the legitimacy of its actions. The ruling conventions of the liberal polity define the limits of public activity, not the formal demands of competing moral theories or the compelling complexities of special cases.

These observations can be seen best in light of a problem that is currently a matter of serious concern at all levels of public policy making in the United States. There seems to be little doubt that in the next generation American society and its government face a very formidable problem regarding the provision of necessary financial support to persons in old age. The declining number of persons entering the work force and the general aging of the baby boom generation, roughly those born between 1945 and 1965, will combine to bankrupt the Social Security system as it is presently constituted and funded sometime in the early decades of the twenty-first century. These facts are not challenged by any serious student of the Social Security system, even those who are staunch defenders of the present system of old-age assistance.[8]

Though the essential features of the long term problem are agreed to on all sides, the solutions are not. The obvious short term solution, tax increases, will probably not be feasible for this longer term problem. Such substantial increases as would be necessary for the long term would certainly lead to deep resentment by those entering the work force and would engender a strong likelihood of undermining necessary incentives for work and productivity. Some solutions calling for Social Security to be merged with the total financing for the federal government and for the resulting deficits to be financed by borrowing as is done for the whole budget will only shift the problem, not solve it. Many other proposals have been made to solve this problem but none has achieved the consensus of support that will be required to enact any substantial changes in the current program of assistance.[9]

One proposal that has not been made, however, is to kill or let die everyone over a certain age. I submit, though, that we could design such a program that would meet every test of consistency and fairness currently endorsed by leading analysts of public policy and leading theories of justice. For example, it is well established that a vastly greater amount of resources goes to the care of the very old, over seventy-five, than would be warranted on the basis of their percentage of the population.[10] These persons are the ones who most frequently cannot provide for their own care and who thus wind up in nursing homes at public expenses. These people are sick more often, more seriously and for longer periods during each illness, all of which adds substantially to the nation's medicare bill. Furthermore, most aged individuals fear death far less than they do the debilitating effects of old age, especially senility.[11]

Why not then put those over seventy-five to death? Such a program would easily solve a serious crisis of the Social Security system. It could easily be established in a fair manner. Everyone over a certain age would be treated equally and the rationale for treating those so situated differently from others could easily be established from a substantial concern for the prudent use of limited resources. It would be consistent, generalizable, and easily understood, the very canons by which contemporary analysts evaluate policy. Moreover it would relieve the suffering of the very old, especially those with chronic debilitating illnesses such as emphysema, and it might eliminate the fear of very old age and senility for the younger citizens. Three of the theories of justice most discussed by contemporary moral theorists could easily be construed to support such a policy. Utilitarian moral theory could certainly be developed in such a fashion as to provide a powerful defense of such a policy. Likewise, moral relativists might also find support for it in the practices of other societies in other settings. Even Rawlsian contract theorists could argue that this resolution is acceptable as a means of preserving a system of assistance that benefits especially the least well off among those who are younger, that is, those who simply could not support themselves without public assistance.

If desired the threshold could be changed from one based on age to one based on disability, though here the required criterion distinguishing those allowed to live from those to be killed would be more difficult to specify, especially with any degree of fairness. For example, it might be concluded that those elderly below a certain level of cognitive functioning and psychomotor ability should be killed. If the level were set properly and adhered to strictly it would be consistent and generalizable and could receive support from some important writers in ethical and policy matters, especially those who now claim that infants with severe disabilities are better off dead.

21

With so much to be said for it, it seems strange that this obvious means of solving an important national problem has not received at least a serious hearing in the court of public opinion. To date it has not, however, and it seems at least as certain as anything that might be said about American society and its government that any proposal of this sort could never be endorsed by the American people. This fact seems so patent and so uncontroversial that we are led to ask why. Why is it that an obvious solution to a pressing problem, that can be justified in so many technically precise ways, is not even open to discussion? Why is the discussion so firmly closed at this point?

The answer can be found in the same place to which Plato points in the dialectical relationship between the regime founded by Socrates in the *Republic* and that founded by the Athenian Stranger in the *Laws:* namely, the concept of a political regime that has its own narrative about how human life ought to be lived, its own principles setting forth the human good and the right derived from that story, its own conventions that embody this good and specific laws to enforce it. Only after this vision is accepted can one meaningfully apply the mathematically based analytical programs that are used by legislators and policy makers to fashion acceptable public policy, a fact that is tacitly admitted by most serious students of public policy and moral philosophy.

It is, of course, the most primeval fact of human existence that human beings live within the governance of distinct political communities. In modern times, however, such a fact has been most frequently conceived of as meaning no more than that human beings must live in different nation-states, each with its own form of government. A regime is thus equated with a form of government and the necessity of human existence in discrete regimes is reduced to a truism.

Understood in this manner, however, crucial features of the existence of human beings in specific political communities are obscured and the study of public matters and policies is distorted. What is obscured is the most essential point, that regimes do not begin as "forms of government," but rather as shared convictions about the good and the just and their proper embodiment in communal life and social norms. Regimes assume a certain vision of the good for human beings and embody that vision in the fundamentally moral choices regarding justice that define their existence as independent human communities, set forth the rights and duties of the rulers and the ruled and establish the various means of enacting, administering and adjudicating the laws.[12] It is this moral choice regarding the human good and the just that brings into being a regime dedicated to those ends and not others. This point can be seen in almost all of the greatest political philosophers of the Western tradition. In this regard, Rousseau's *Poland* is an especially penetrating text. In it he shows the careful dialectic that develops between convention and change in regimes. Rousseau would both preserve Poland as an entity and change it as a regime by preserving the outward forms of Polish life and institutions and instituting fundamental changes in the principles that animate the civic life of the Poles.[13]

This understanding of a regime or political community enables us to give an account of things that seem obvious to common observation but which cannot be grasped fully when the terms of understanding are limited to social systems or forms of government. Even the most untrained observer knows that the Iranian regime underwent a fundamental transformation when the Ayatollah Khomeni assumed the power which the shah once held completely. This is true even though the general structures of each regime are in significant ways remarkably similar. In each case contemporary thought classifies them as authoritarian regimes, with political power concentrated in the hands of one leader or a small group of leaders, with a secret police operating in extralegal ways at the behest of these leaders, with punishment also meted out in extralegal, even terroristic ways. Even more obvious to most observers is the difference between Stalinist Russia and the new revolutionary regime in Iran, although the similarities as authoritarian governments are, if anything, more marked than those noted in a comparison with the rule of the shah. Looked at in another case, the similarities between the political and social life of the United States and Great Britain are obvious to the most un-

schooled observer, although their differences in form of government are at least as marked as those that differentiate revolutionary Iran and the Soviet Union.

This view can be seen even within the United States itself.
For example, every serious observer of politics in the various
states knows that Utah is a "Mormon" state and that political
life in Utah is dominated by the "Mormon" religion. To note
only the most obvious point, almost all of the senators, gover-
nors, and congressmen from Utah have had firm roots in Mormon soil. Yet the form of government in Utah is equivalent to
that which is found in other states and the various constitutional guarantees concerning the separation of church and state are,
if anything, more faithfully observed. Conceived of as a whole,
the political community of Utah is dominated by the Mormon
faith but this fact will not come to life if our focus is on forms of
government nor even on the issues discussed in state politics
for they are the same issues that trouble other states: environmental concerns, welfare, educational support, resource con-
servation, and the like.[14]

In each of these instances, the differences or similarities
common sense perceives come to light in full fashion only
when we grasp the difference between a regime and a form of
government. Regimes start with a shared commitment to some
end, some idea of the good for man and a belief in how the
political community can be brought to serve that end. The
difference between pre- and post-revolutionary Iran, for example, lies in the importance attached to the Islamic religion and
its legal codes in defining the human good and its means of
realization. From this follows the certainty of the rulers, who
follow not their own whims but the will of God, who allow no
real debates because they believe that God allows none, who
govern in an authoritarian manner because God and his representatives must not be challenged, and who enjoy broad
support from a population that is largely devout.[15] In all of
these specific instances and in much more subtle ways, a set
of opinions about human good establishes the terms within
which political life is carried on, the issues of importance, the

manner of their discussion, and the proper range of alternative solutions.

As can be seen in Utah, the centrality of these choices regarding the good and the just appears even in cases where the institutional forms of governance are essentially the same as those found elsewhere. Despite the formal equivalence of the institutions of political life, one searches in vain for another state identified as is Utah by a specific religion which dominates the lives of its citizens and the political life of the state. For example, one searches largely in vain for another state in which ratification of the Equal Rights Amendment simply was not an issue of political controversy. The dominant religion decided to oppose ratification; the matter was closed. In the same way, were it not for the Supreme Court decision, the question of liberalized abortion law would not have been a salient political issue—as it is, Utah is a source of strong anti-abortion sentiment.

The choice regarding the good and the just is coeval with the existence of the regime itself. Having made such a choice, regimes implicitly reject the fundamental alternatives with which their own organizing principles cannot be reconciled. In other words, the regime both articulates in its way of life an opinion regarding the good and the just and closes off the horizon of choice among the alternatives. The questions regarding those alternatives are closed questions for political practice within the regime itself. To raise such questions is to raise the question of the justice of the regime itself and thus of its claim to embody an understanding of justice that merits the commitment of its citizens.[16]

Viewed in this manner, no regime is or can be the utterly open society made famous in the writings of some contemporary philosophers and civil libertarians.[17] The society in which all questions are open questions is a construct, intellectually tantalizing but false to reality and impossible in practice. It may even be dangerous to attempt to do so since it diverts attention from the humanly possible and just alternatives. No matter how much personal liberty and inquisitiveness the liberal regime can permit, in policy and law it still must impose answers to those questions regarding the justice of the regime itself, the very regime that permits wide liberty of thought and action. Any regime can sustain itself over time only to the extent that it remembers these fundamental truths. Regimes sustain themselves by sustaining the conventions of public belief and commitment that essentially distinguish the regime itself. Even liberal regimes can safely dedicate themselves to the widest possible degree of personal liberty only when that liberty is sustained and given direction by principles which are themselves outside the matrix of free inquiry and action which they protect.[18]

Aristotlean Observation and Analysis

Though now displaced in favor of the language of systems analysis,[19] this understanding of political regimes returns us to the classical sources of the political philosophy of the West. The most developed and penetrating articulation of this understanding is found in Aristotle's *Politics*. This is not obvious to the casual American reader because existing British translations fundamentally obscure Aristotle's teaching for them by translating the key term *politeia* sometimes as *form of government* and at other times as *constitution*.[20] Both of these are part of any regime, but they mislead in identifying the less essential part as the core phenomena. The problems with a form of government formulation have just been noted. The constitution formulation is somewhat closer to the mark, if *unwritten* is understood. Indeed, the founding documents of any regime may be expected to give written articulation to the concept of justice which animates its civic life; nevertheless, no such written document can define the whole way of life of a community as can the ruling opinions regarding justice and virtue—these opinions define much more than merely the formation and arrangement of the offices of government and the rights of citizens. A written constitution is a legal phenomenon which prescinds from the core of the regime itself. The interpretation of *politeia* as *constitution* with no qualification may divert attention from the regime itself to the secondary phenomenon of the government and its organization and thus back to the form-of-government formulation as this form is described in the constitution.

But a close attention to Aristotle's discussion and the nuances of his language helps us to avoid these problems and gain a deeper understanding of the relation between regime and government. Aristotle's famous sixfold division of governmental forms is premised not on whether the one, the few, or the many rule, but on the different conceptions of justice that each government embodies and which legitimate rule by the one, the few or the many.[21] Oligarchy and democracy for example differ precisely because of differing beliefs as to what it is that confers equality and inequality and hence what legitimates the ruler. From these differences follow different laws and constitutions that enshrine wealth, property, or free birth as the measure of citizenship.

As Aristotle notes, regimes differ in the way they arrange the different parts, especially participation in the governing of the regime. But these differences of division follow from an opinion regarding the proper or just principle of division, that is, what it is that constitutes the just basis for assigning the tasks of governance among the various parts. Even the subtypes of various regimes may be distinguished by the degree to which they adhere to the principle of justice inherent in the species itself, or depart from it in varying degrees. A democratic regime in which poor and rich are counted alike, equally sovereign and equally impotent acting alone, is closest in spirit to the concept of justice implicit in democracy itself.[22] A democratic regime that permits participation on the basis of property qualifications is to be distinguished precisely because of its premise regarding justice. In such a regime all free men are not actually equal in political rights. Though participation is sufficiently broadly based to enable the regime to be classed as democratic, the division of its parts differs because its conception of justice differs from that found in the purer forms of democracy.[23]

From the fundamental conception of justice which defines democratic regimes flow the other features of democracy and the way of life peculiar in democratic societies. For example, Aristotle notes that democratic regimes are based on the rule of law. At one point he appears to teach that the rule of law is part of any regime but his discussion of monarchy shows that his true teaching is that the rule of law is part of any practical regime, especially any regime in which the many rule.[24]

What he demonstrates is the necessary connection between democratic regimes and the rule of law. In democratic societies the many are the ultimate source of governing authority. But the great mass of people have neither the leisure nor the temperament to decide matters of governance and justice with the consistency and frequency required for political life. Hence they establish the superiority of law as a means of setting forth a permanent standard of public justice. This is an imperfect standard of justice, as Aristotle well knows. Given the nature of democratic societies, however, it is the only standard available. The alternatives either take us out of the confines of public justice or transcend the necessary limits of democratic rule.[25]

In this regard we might note Aristotle's famous discussion of *epieikeia*, often translated as *equity*. In both the *Nichomachean Ethics* and the *Politics*, this is said to be a species of virtue that enables one to apply inflexible legal rules to specific cases in which they may only partially apply or where the case at hand may be the exception where following the rule leads to greater injustice.[26]

However desirable it may be to temper legal justice with equity in this fashion, such tempering poses serious problems for practice, especially democratic practice. Unless we wish to destroy the rule itself, we need to know the proper limits of equity. Otherwise, each one becomes the judge of his or her case, and public judgment becomes impossible. But the knowledge thus required by the equity principle transcends the limits of the law and thus the limits of the democratic principle, namely, when the law should be obeyed and when not. This, of course, is the foundation not of democracy but aristocracy and the possibility of such knowledge is something which democratic regimes must publicly deny. We shall return to this matter in the next chapter when we discuss democratic regimes in more detail. Here it is sufficient to note that Aristotle's most famous discussion of equity appears not in the *Politics* at all but in the *Ethics*, a work which does not purport to offer a political teaching and which is not directed to the many who are the source of democratic rule.[27] In the *Politics*, however, the discussion of equity is limited to the question of whether monarchy is the best form of government and the precise relationship of such a regime to the rule of law. Specifically the concept of equity is never mentioned in the discussion of democratic regimes.[28] We also note that Aristotle's discussion of equity and political justice in the *Rhetoric* gives three sorts of cases in which equity is called for; none of these raises the most central issues for democratic practice. One is where the case is not covered by the law, that is, where the legislator has left a gap which the court or administrator must fill in. The other cases are those in which the legislator cannot enumerate all of the possible cases in statutory law owing either to the complexity of the subject or the number of instances involved. These situations require one to prescind from the rule to the case, in an intuitive fashion. What is silently ignored, however, is precisely the instance where one knows that the case is clearly covered by the rule but one believes on some other grounds that the rule ought to be set aside here because justice lies elsewhere. This is the very case that, if generally admitted, would evacuate the rule of law as a meaningful concept and is especially troubling in democratic regimes which consciously foster individual interests, passions and biases.[29]

In this regard, Aristotle also notes that democratic regimes ostracize or banish those of superior abilities, wealth or political influence because their presence in political life cannot be squared with the democratic principle. Thus democratic regimes both embody a particular conception of justice and exclude the fundamental alternatives as a matter of law. Since the alternatives are so fundamental that they cannot coexist, one must give. To admit them both is to have the proverbial house divided. To admit the cogency of the monarchial or oligarchal principle is to admit that democracy is unjust and therefore unworthy of allegiance and sacrifice on its behalf, something which no regime can do in practice. Of course, Aristotle notes, a man of extraordinary virtue ought to be accorded the power of governance; viewed by this standard banishing such a man is unjust. But it is required by the demands of democratic rule and thus, as a matter of practice, becomes just in democratic terms.[30]

Aristotle says much more about the nature and construction of democratic regimes but we have seen enough for our purposes. He works out the practical significance of a given understanding of justice as embodied in the organizing principles of a certain sort of regime, showing what it excludes as well as how it organizes the regime and forms the ultimate context within which any substantive policy must be judged.

This understanding of the most important political fact is carried forward in Aristotle's discussion of drastic political change, or what we now loosely call *revolutions*. The essence of such drastic change is a transformation in the ruling opinions regarding justice and it is because some men come to desire another form of justice in practice that they become revolutionaries. Thus the precise form of government or the exact makeup of the ruling body is not central in the study of political change or development, especially drastic change. To be sure, institutional forms do point to these more central phenomena of change and development, a fact which Aristotle stresses repeatedly. But these are not the heart of the matter and attention directed at institutional change is necessarily diverted away from these more fundamental aspects of political change.[31]

In order for us to gain a proper understanding of the most comprehensive of political phenomena, the regime, Aristotle directs our attention to the features coeval with its existence. From these central features he shows how the legislator or founder could devise institutional forms and laws compatible with it. In a substantial number of instances, there will likely be a range of options for the legislator each at least not incompatible with the defining characteristics of the regime. These are the limits of a proper choice. Beyond these limits of the regime itself are those choices that embody a fundamentally different conception of the just and the good and thus imply a fundamentally different sort of regime. For the legislator proper, as opposed to the founder, these choices are closed.

30

Aristotle's analysis is much richer and more profound than anything that can be said here. He directs our attention to that comprehensive point from which all law and policy ultimately flow and to which such law and policy must bear a consistent and derivative relationship. Law and policy do not exist *de novo*, in a vacuum constructed of whim, caprice, or abstract morality. They exist in the context of specific regimes, animated by different organizing principles, with citizens of differing capacities for civic virtue, differing moral sentiments and with differing racial, linguistic, geographic, economic, and social divisions and characteristics. In the context of these differences, the legislator seeks to bring to light in law and policy the concept of justice inherent in the regime itself and thus perfect the whole by better realizing the latent characteristics in its parts.

To understand policy is thus to understand the regime itself and the requirements of its governance in any given circumstance. It is not, therefore, possible to equate a proper understanding of policy and the requirements of its study with a correct understanding of mathematical tools of analysis or with the results of using such tools. Mathematics is simply incapable of expressing the discriminations necessary for public life. These differentiations only come into view in light of the regime itself and its ruling conceptions of the just and the good. A regime is not a mathematical construct. Mathematics is blind to the regime. In modern parlance it is a neutral means of expressing relationships among variables. But precisely because of its supposed neutrality, fascination with mathematics is the most alluring error of policy analysis. Since it cannot teach us about the regime itself or express in its terms the choices that define the regime, its influence is not therefore neutral regarding the connection between regimes and policies. In diverting attention away from that relationship, it suggests that policy and law are less important than they are and that the usual methods of policy analysis and evaluation are more significant than they may be. But this either locates the making of truly decisive political choices elsewhere or ignores them altogether. In either case, the tasks of the one who must make such public decisions are rendered fundamentally obscure.

31

For our purpose we have concentrated attention on Aristotle's discussion of democratic regimes and the manner in which this brings to light the central features of his teaching on the nature of political regimes and their relation to the laws and institutions that take shape in them. Aristotle, however, also illuminates the practical import of this teaching in his discussion of actual regimes in book two of the *Politics*. The best example of this is his examination of Sparta. He begins by noting that the Spartan regime is founded upon a specific commitment to one form of goodness, namely, military prowess. As a result, Sparta was unequaled as a battlefield combatant. But though they knew how to win a war, they perpetually lost the peace. By concentrating on military pursuits and the forms of rule appropriate to a conquering army, they were diverted from learning the art of governing well their own regime where peace, not war and conquest must be the goal. Hence, some extraordinarily defective practices flowered in the regime itself, precisely because those who ought to have ruled properly were either off at war or diverted by planning and preparations for war when at home.

The fundamental defects in the Spartan regime are not those of particular leaders or institutional forms. Rather they stem from the ruling conception of the good which is, itself, defective and thus gives rise to defective leadership and political institutions. Such a defective conception of the good permits the emergence of those institutional and social defects that in turn destroy the effectiveness of the regime even in time of battle, since any military involvement will require an effective domestic regime to support it if it is to be successful in its adventures.[32]

De Tocqueville's Critique of American Democratic Society

The Aristotlean understanding of regimes as communities of belief and commitment, and the requirements of their governance, is developed at length in what is perhaps the most profound examination of a specific regime undertaken in modern times: Alexis de Tocqueville's analysis of American democratic society. His examination of the American political community is far too rich and comprehensive for us to pretend to undertake any truly adequate analysis of it here. Yet we can call attention to the manner in which de Tocqueville demonstrates how the ruling opinions and conventions of the American regime work themselves out in policies, practices, and social forms.[33] For this purpose we might have chosen any of a very wide number of practices or public conventions such as constitutional forms or the absence of property qualifications for voting which de Tocqueville discusses with precision and insight.[34] In each case he shows how the fundamental democratic commitment to equality shapes and gives direction to the policies and practices that take root in American life. Perhaps the most interesting example of this pervasive function of the belief in equality comes not in the more obvious or more political contexts. Rather it comes in his discussion of the place of organized religion and religious beliefs in American life and their relation to the American regime. In essence he shows how the fundamental democratic belief in equality shapes the practice of religion in America and in turn is moderated and given a foundation by the popular religiousness of the American people.[35]

In America the fundamental conviction of equality which founds the regime both includes those religious forms and opinions that are compatible and even necessary to its success and excludes those that are not. Religious opinions that cannot be squared with the convictions that found the regime are reduced to silence or relegated to insignificant sectarian backwaters. So much is this the case that, de Tocqueville claims, "all clergy speak the same language," at least on fundamental questions that lie at the core of the vision in which the regime defines its existence.[36] De Tocqueville surely knew that our various denominations differed immensely among themselves on matters which they regarded as significant for the salvation of man. Though the various denominations may have considered with the utmost seriousness such matters as the precise composition of the Trinity or the exact nature of the eternal

33

punishments meted out to the wicked, it can hardly be claimed that such questions touch on the convictions that define the community itself and embody its distinct sense of the good and the just. In matters that do touch on these foundational opinions, religion itself becomes democratized in both form and content as the examples of various protestant denominations and even Roman Catholicism demonstrates.[37]

This point is best illustrated by the example of Roman Catholicism whose practices de Tocqueville knew intimately as an adherent. Roman Catholicism, particularly in the nineteenth century, had grown up in circumstances that were often hostile to and at best uninterested in democratic regimes. It was thus often supposed that the Catholic Church and its faithful members were at best lukewarm democrats. This, de Tocqueville strenuously argued, was not so. Whatever may have been true of the Catholicism of Metternich and de Maistre, who were bitter enemies of democracy, in America Catholicism spoke the same democratic language as did its protestant brethren.[38] Insofar as form is concerned, Catholicism partook of the same general spirit of informality of religious practice in America which, for one schooled in the heavily liturgical religious life of Europe was a striking departure: "I have seen no country in which Christianity is less clothed in forms, symbols and observances than it is in the United States. . . . This is true of Roman Catholics as well as of other beliefs. Nowhere else do Catholic priests show so little taste for petty individual observances, for extraordinary and peculiar ways to salvation, and nowhere else do they care so much for the spirit and so little for the letter of the law."[39]

De Tocqueville argues that it is precisely these sorts of ornate religious observances that direct people to concern themselves primarily with ultimately divisive and inegalitarian religious convictions; my way becomes the only way to salvation; unless you practice the way I do, worship at my altar, and pay homage to my saints you can expect nothing but damnation from God. Such religious forms and practices are patently inegalitarian and in America they are, for the most part, either

34

ignored or reduced to insignificance, insofar as the things that matter most in religious life are concerned.

The content of religious belief is even more strikingly altered by the democratic conviction concerning equality. In America, de Tocqueville notes, one simply did not hear the view of the Roma Curia that "error, (that is, religious error) has no rights." Such an opinion is a frank denial of the notion of the civil equality of religious opinions which constitutes one of the founding principles of the American polity. Even more significant for de Tocqueville is the manner in which the content of religious belief is silently reduced in the minds of the many to the sorts of propositions that all sincere religious believers, especially Christian believers can find acceptable. "Nowhere else is the mind fed with clearer, simpler or more comprehensive conceptions. Though American Christians are divided into very many sects they all see their religion in the same light."[40] Except in its sectarian forms, American religious communities and clergymen preach to their congregations the simple religious truths that are widely shared, egalitarian in their import, and limited to matters of central religious significance, not to matters of social order and political practice in which religious belief can be divisive and inegalitarian. "Religion in America is a world apart in which the clergyman is supreme but one in which he is careful never to leave. Within its limits he guides men's minds while outside them he leaves them to themselves."[41]

If the egalitarian impulse of democratic regimes ultimately shapes the practice of religion in these communities, so too does religion itself shape democratic life in necessary and beneficial ways. This occurs in two ways. On the one hand, the conventions of democratic regimes unleash an anarchy of political opinions, each equally justified by its being firmly held by some group of citizens, however small. On the other hand they also breed an acquisitiveness born of the lack of any conviction regarding a natural social order in which the individual finds one's place. Since all men are equal, all can equally pursue material well-being through self interested commercial endeavors. But this intellectual anarchy and rampant selfishness render it difficult for human beings to believe in anything very firmly or to sacrifice for the larger good of the community and its well-being. The restless, selfish individual which de Tocqueville saw as characteristic of democratic regimes, was, he believed, very limited in the capacity for patriotism or courage on behalf of others, both of which the community requires if even the rights to guarantee individual liberty to pursue material wealth are to be preserved.

Popular religiousness moderates these deficiencies in the democratic impulse but only insofar as it adopts a democratic form and fundamentally democratic opinions. By supplying some answers to the common man regarding one's immortal soul and its future state, answers that are compatible with the democratic view of the good and the just, it averts the danger that the many will seek ultimate satisfaction in this life through demagoguery; by teaching human beings to tame their selfish passions in the direction of concern for others, it renders communal life humane and just, and enables the proper defense of the regime from its enemies.

The religiousness of the American people, however, is no accident. That Americans are substantially more enamored of organized religious forms and observances than are Europeans is a fact admitted by every serious student of the subject, including de Tocqueville himself.[42] For de Tocqueville this was a direct result of the leveling of political opinion engendered by the attachment to equality. Human beings cannot remain without some beliefs that they regard as ultimate or absolute, to which they give unquestioning allegiance.[43] In modern psychological language, this is said to be the need to believe in something that will give one's life meaning. For this purpose the individual can either bind himself or herself to a political opinion and thus prepare oneself for absolute, slave-like obedience to whoever purports to govern on the basis of that opinion or one can find this meaning in the context of religious opinions about God and the human soul.[44] The triumph of the democratic regime and its ruling opinions renders the former alternative dangerous and leads directly to a specifically democratic form of religiousness which moderates and perfects the democratic regime by answering to this need for meaning and providing the psychological resources for courage, sacrifice and patriotism by citizens.[45]

In his examination of the American regime's expression of democratic principles, de Tocqueville constantly notes what these principles either exclude or include as acceptable institutional forms and public policies. Sometimes he explicitly contrasts American conventions and laws with the aristocratic and oligarchic regimes of Europe; his experience of both enabled him to see fundamental political alternatives in a clearer light. Often he does it by implication as in the discussion of the laws regarding inheritance, which in the United States deliberately preclude the formation of great landed estates that form the basis of these aristocratic and oligarchic regimes. By seeing the regime in light of the fundamental alternatives that confront it, de Tocqueville deepens the understanding of the regime itself as a whole and the proper arrangement of its various parts, both those arrangements engendered by its ruling beliefs and conventions and those arrangements and alternatives excluded by these same commitments.

Having enriched our understanding of the most comprehensive of political phenomena, the regime, we are prepared to return to the practical inquiry with which we began: namely, how can we properly begin to examine serious matters of public policy and choice, especially ones that cannot really be adequately addressed in the quantitative manner in which most public policy is examined. Such sciences are of use only when the choices faced by the legislator or policy maker can be adequately expressed in quantitative terms. As a result, the proper employment of such means of evaluation requires a more comprehensive understanding of when the alternatives presented for consideration can be fully expressed in the terms required for these methods of analysis. To employ the techniques properly, therefore, is to transcend them.

This transcendence occurs in the first instance, through a proper understanding of the regime within which policy is to be formed. Such understanding illuminates the nature of the choices faced by the legislator both by leading to reflection on the manner in which any proposed alternative will cohere with the principles defining the regime itself and by implicitly limiting the choices one may actually consider to those consistent with the ruling premise of the regime. Having understood the nature of the regime and the form of justice that constitutes its ruling convictions, the legislator can gain the necessary insight into the choices that present themselves for public decision. One can see which issues are properly resolved by government in such a polity, and which alternative resolutions are rendered illegitimate by such a regime. The legislator is prepared to see which of the practically available alternatives best meet the needs of citizens in this regime, which do so only in a partial or tangential manner, and which will actually be harmful, given the nature of the regime and the specific virtues it nourishes in its citizens.

On this basis, we can answer the queries which initiated our search for a comprehensive point of departure for the consideration of alternative public policies: what is wrong with the proposed solution to the crisis in Social Security funding and why has such a solution not received a serious hearing when other patently insufficient solutions have? A complete grasp of such a proposal necessitates a fuller understanding of our regime, which is developed in the next chapter. We can briefly anticipate the results of that discussion here as a means of illustrating the significance of the results of our inquiry so far.

Liberal democratic regimes begin with the belief in the equal worth of every human being, from whence they derive a commitment to individual liberty. Since no one is so superior that he or she ought to rule, everyone has the equal right to rule. This is the foundation of the claim of the many to rule and hence of both democratic government and the liberty of the individual from one's fellow citizens who have no just claim to rule of themselves. This belief in the equal worth of each human being, at least in politically decisive terms, is made possible by a deliberate diminution of those aspects of human goodness relevant for political choice to the needs of a man as a physiological entity. In liberal theory the proper ends of the

38

political regime become reduced to the preservation of human life. That is, the rights to life, liberty and property become central, with the latter justified in terms of the former.[46]

This claim about equal worth and its corollary, the equal right to life, is deeply embedded in our law and custom which treats the killing of the derelict on par with the murder of a saint. In terms of such a ruling belief, we can understand the proffered solution to the problem of old-age assistance as one which transcends the principles which define the regime itself. It would require us to designate one group of citizens, as no longer bearers of the equal and inalienable right to life. It is not that it would require transgressing a constitutional right. The constitution could be amended if necessary. What the common revulsion against such a policy points to is a correct, though perhaps untutored perception that such a policy simply cannot be squared with the organizing principles of the regime and thus with the foundation of the constitution itself.

Furthermore, democratic regimes foster both a selfish acquisitiveness in their citizens and a sentiment of compassion toward others. By treating all as equal, it opens up the common man to the possibility of satisfying one's material desires by one's own effort—hence the profoundly acquisitive character of democratic citizens. However, by reducing each individual to the level of one's fellows and liberating one from the bonds of custom and class, such regimes turn man's attention to one's own weakness as well. Because all desires cannot be satisfied the liberation of such desires inevitably leads to unhappiness. Moreover, by turning man's attention to the similarities he or she bears with his or her fellows it engenders a sense of commonality, a feeling that all are in the same boat together; such is the ease with which democratic man imagines himself as being beset with the misfortunes of another. "There but for the grace of God go I" is a quintessential lament of the democratic citizen.[47]

The tension between acquisitiveness and compassion lies at the heart of many of our most explosive public issues. A proper discussion of the just means of resolving that tension lies outside the confines of this book. We may note here that both in theory and in practice our regime seems unable to accept for very long a public policy that explicitly resolves this tension in a manner inconsistent with the premises of the regime, and thus also inconsistent with the proper claims of both parts of this tension. It seems clear on inspection, however, that the proffered solution to the problem of old age assistance is just such a solution. This realization enables us to understand the complete silence among the American people regarding such a policy. The proffered policy can be squared with neither the premises of the regime nor with the moral sentiments that those premises nourish in the citizenry. Except in exceptional circumstances legislators cannot and should not be expected to transcend the limits of the regime and the people themselves cannot be expected to acquiesce for long in policies that violate their deepest moral sentiments.

A further examination of the defining premises of liberal democratic regimes will occupy us in the next chapter. The results of our inquiry to date indicate that a proper analysis of the specific issues that concern us cannot begin without such an examination. What we have seen so far is that those attempts to provide the means of examining and evaluating public issues that do not begin with an understanding of the regime within which policy is formed are at best incomplete. These methods seem incapable of even adequately explaining obvious facts such as the silence of the American people regarding any method of solving problems of old age assistance like that described at the outset of this chapter. This chapter will have served its purposes if it has demonstrated the need for the inquiry to which we now turn as a necessary precondition for considering the specific issues treated later.

CHAPTER TWO

Liberal Polities

Introduction

The political regimes of the modern West, in this instance especially the American regime, derive their inspiration from the teachings of the founders of modern political philosophy, chiefly Hobbes and Locke and those who followed them, such as Rousseau and Kant. The transformation of political thought and action brought about under the inspiration of these writers was substantive and fundamental in its break with classical political philosophy. To understand the nature of modern regimes is to understand this transformation.[1]

The political regimes founded in the wake of this transformation have often been called *liberal* or *democratic* regimes. Of course, this is only a general title used to denote a group of regimes that are founded on fundamentally similar or equivalent organizing principles.[2] Whether this title or some other is used is not essential, though for reasons of convenience and continuity with an ongoing tradition of inquiry I have chosen to use the term *liberal regimes*. The crucial point is that the regimes of the modern West are founded on certain core principles which are coeval with the existence of liberal democratic polities. These premises define the existence of this sort of regime and mark the threshold of entering into the class itself. Our examination into the core premises on which liberal regimes are founded will require a careful, if necessarily brief, inquiry into the roots of these regimes and the works of their greatest expositors, defenders and founders. From these sources we may gain some understanding of the principles on which liberal, free regimes are founded and without which they cannot be sustained.

Liberal Critique of Classical Political Regimes

At the core of liberalism lies a seminal critique of classical political philosophy and the regimes animated by its guiding spirit. This critique centered on the problem of human excellence or virtue, and especially on its relation to political rule. For the ancients the fundamental given of political life was the natural right of the wise and virtuous to rule over those less well endowed with the characteristics of human excellence. Variations on this fundamental point can be found in every political philosopher of consequence in Western thought before the Renaissance, that is, before Marsilius and Machiavelli. As Plato says, "The man with real knowledge, the true statesman, will in many instances allow his actions to be dictated by his art and pay no regard to written prescriptions."[3] Correspondingly, the fundamental political problem was how to design a regime in which this sort of natural justice might flourish over time and in which men might be molded to the demanding standard of excellence in virtue of wisdom. Both Plato and Aristotle, of course, realized that a perfectly just regime was not possible, given the imperfections of human beings and the limitations imposed by climate, geography, international relations, and so forth. The implications of this realization are profound and will be noted in due course. It does not alter, however, the essence of the classical belief that true natural right was based on human excellence and that natural justice required a political re-

42

gime in which excellence ruled and re-created itself over time.

From Machiavelli and Hobbes onward, modern political philosophers have stood this view on its head. They rejected both the proposition concerning human excellence and the proposition that perfectly just political rule was founded on such excellence to begin with and ought to foster its continuous development. Virtue was no longer regarded either as the proper end of political life or as the precondition of the true right to rule.[4] The founders of liberalism deliberately forsook the pursuit of virtue in the classical sense in favor of a regime dedicated to the widest possible measure of liberty of the individual to pursue private ends which may be immoral or dubiously moral. The founders were concerned foremost to establish a regime "conceived in liberty," committed not to the education of the individual for a supposed higher virtue, but to individual choice based on private estimates of what is valuable. Hence, Rawls, for example, can dismiss almost without serious argument any "higher virtue" theory of justice, as being incompatible with the conventional opinions of liberal regimes.[5] Rawls's critics are both correct on justice proper, which indeed requires a concept of higher virtue, and wrong on the conventions of liberalism.[6] This point is more complex than can be addressed here, but it is essentially correct for the liberal tradition as a whole.[7]

Viewed from this perspective, the regime itself has no purpose beyond assuring that an individual's pursuit of his private goals does not unreasonably infringe on either the requirements for the preservation of the regime itself or the similar and equally plausible pursuit of other ends by other individuals. Thus truncated, the realm of politics came to center chiefly on the needs of human beings as physiological entities, as bodies in classical terminology.[8] Political man had been stripped of his soul, so to speak, and was left as a biological organism who had the additional ability of being able to pursue distant and often fanciful objectives. This abstraction from the human soul and its virtue left political man equal with his fellows as a physiological being and, in essence, rendered the assertion of equality *vis-à-vis* the ends of politics as the *sine qua non* of liberal regimes.

43

This rejection of classical political philosophy has two moments in liberal theory, one epistemic and the other prudential. First, many modern philosophers were skeptical of claims to know the nature of human excellence in any definitive way. For some philosophers such historicist or positivist skepticism of value claims led directly to nihilism. Secondly, there was a profound distrust of anyone who claimed to have a definitive grasp on the meaning of human excellence. From Hobbes and Spinoza onward, both kinds of skepticism exercised a powerful influence on liberal theory. If no one really knows, in a decisive manner, what constitutes human excellence, either because there is no such standard or because it is impossible to know it, then a politics based on such claims must be fundamentally unjust.[9]

More important, the founders of liberalism profoundly distrusted a politics based on such claims to knowledge. Even granting that such knowledge existed and that a very few might possess it, they regarded it as extremely doubtful that such men would be able to exercise a position of political power for very long. Unrestrained power in the hands of the wise eventually degenerated into unrestrained power with none of the moderating virtues of moral or intellectual excellence that prevented it from becoming mere tyranny. As devout students of the classics, the founders of liberalism well knew that Periclean Athens quickly degenerated to the point where the truly wise man was executed by the city. The brilliance of Augustus was soon followed by the likes of Nero and Caligula, each wielding the same power as did their illustrious predecessor. Even Augustus was far from being the paradigm of human excellence which classical political philosophy required for perfectly just, absolute political rule. As a matter of prudence, therefore, the assertion of an absolute right to rule as a result of superior human virtue was in fact dangerous. It was far more likely to legitimate the pretentions of tyrants than to establish in power those truly fit to rule by reason of excellence.

Liberal theory thus came to view man from the bottom up. He was a biological entity; anything more was irrelevant to political man. To assert anything more was seen as asserting a politically decisive difference among men that was both difficult to justify and dangerous to practice. The politically decisive category was the category of the species, human being. Everything else paled in importance. The fundamental lines to be drawn for political practice were those between man and the divine on the one hand and between man and the animals on the other. In between all human beings are equal in their worth, in the rights which they bear in relation to themselves, their fellows and the regime in which they find themselves. They are also, therefore, equal in the fundamental obligations which they have *vis-à-vis* each other, namely the obligation to respect the rights of others.

Postulate of Equality

At this point we must face the core premise of liberal theory: the belief in human equality. From this premise everything flows in liberal political philosophy. Deny it and liberal, democratic regimes cannot be sustained. Human equality is the postulate that every significant theoretician of liberal regimes from the beginning of the modern era to the present articulated. It is the premise from which liberal, free government is derived in Hobbes, Locke, Rousseau, Kant, the Federalist, Jefferson, Lincoln and scores of lesser luminaries, or modern theorists.

None of these philosophers and statesmen, not even the essential theorists of modern political philosophy, ever undertake to demonstrate that man is equal in the politically decisive sense of equal moral standing or dignity. Some of them, it is true, refer to the fact that all human beings are equal with respect to their basic bodily needs and in their aversion to pain, that is, they are equal as physiological entities. But this can hardly ground any claim about political equality or equal rights, which are the decisive forms of equality in liberal thought and practice. In the writings of the founders of liberalism, this sort of equality occurs not as something to be proven, but, rather as something assumed. Jefferson called it self-evident, but this hides the real truth.[10] It is not self-evident in any usual sense.

45

What is empirically self-evident is inequality in physical strength, intellectual prowess, virtuous habits of character and thousands of other characteristics of human beings. The language of *self-evidence* obscures the true nature of equality as a postulate, a necessary premise of free government. As the language of self-evidence suggests, this postulate is not to be proven, at least not in the manner of an empirical proposition. Equality in the politically meaningful or decisive sense is not a scientific proposition, it is a moral postulate. It is an assumption from which liberal regimes can be fashioned and without which they cannot.

Though this understanding of equality is found in all of the core thinkers of modern political philosophy, it is most clearly visible in Hobbes and Locke, from whence it finds its way into Rousseau, Kant, and the American Founding Fathers; thus it became, as Tocqueville and Lincoln knew, both the essential premise of the American regime and the most pervasive convention of the American public creed.

Locke begins his derivation of the liberal regime by positing the doctrine of human equality. It is, he says, a self-evident proposition and he proceeds to quote the "judicious Hooker" for support in this belief.[11] Hooker, however, does not prove that men are equal any more than Locke does. Hooker regards it simply as self-evident and "beyond question." Significantly, Hooker does not derive political implications of the sort Locke does from the presumption of equality. In the passage to which Locke refers, Hooker argues that since men are equal, one has the same natural duty of love towards one's fellows that one has towards oneself.[12] This, of course, is one form of the Christian golden rule and Hooker so interprets it, as a moral rule given by "natural reason." While interesting, this derivation from the premise of equality is hardly the same as that in Locke where equality is source of a right to preserve oneself, not a duty to preserve others. For Locke equality is the engine that forces one to recognize that others have these same rights and thus to realize the necessity of forming a common government that can protect the right of all.[13]

In the discussion of equality, Locke pays lip service to the

46

notion that "creatures of the same species and rank presumably born to all the same faculties should also be equal one amongst another." But this is little more than a tautology. Locke knows full well that some men are stronger or smarter or more cunning than others. They are not all "born to the same advantages of nature" and in this sense they are patently unequal. In fact it is this very inequality that forces men to form political regimes to protect themselves from those whose greater prowess would permit them to invade the rights and plunder the property of the many without hindrance. In the crucial sense, therefore, equality is a moral premise. For Locke men are equal insofar as their moral standing is concerned. They are equal in their worth and hence in their rights. The idea of human equality reduces to a belief that men are equal in their moral standing as human beings, a crucial but essentially unprovable proposition that is the core of Locke's teaching at this point.[14]

In this regard it is important to examine carefully Locke's discussion of man's position in the state of nature. The centerpiece of this is his treatment of the right of punishment in the state of nature. Essentially Locke concludes that, in the state of nature, each man may punish transgressions of the law of nature—that is, every man may punish transgressions of his rights. The anarchic violence to which such a right gives rise is the source of the crucial necessity to form a political regime which will bring order out of this chaos. Never once, however, does Locke suggest that all men are able to punish violations of their rights, or even that they will all desire to do so. The whole discussion is couched in terms of what individuals have an equal right to do. Their vastly differing abilities to exercise such a right are silently ignored.[15]

From the equality of human beings thus conceived, Locke derives liberal government. The equal moral standing of the individual means that no man is so superior in his standing that he can or ought to rule as a matter of right, nor is one so superior in wisdom and virtue that he may justly violate the rights of others with impunity, as God is said to be permitted to do on some theological premises. The equal standing of all generates to equal right of all to a government that respects that doctrine of individual rights, flows from the premise of equality. Without such a premise political liberty is indefensible in principle, for then one man or group would have a right to rule in virtue of his superior standing. By denying that anyone had such a standing Locke breaks with the ancients and makes a regime based on popular will a just and sustainable alternative.

In Hobbes this same sort of maneuver first appeared with only superficial differences from Locke. Hobbes begins his discussion by suggesting that human beings are "so equal" in "the faculties of the body" that the "difference between man and man" is not "so considerable as that one man can thereupon claim for himself any benefit to which another may not pretend as well as he."[16] This is deceptively simple and ambiguous. He does not really claim that men are physically equal. What he says is that men are equal "enough," so that their claims to material possession are equal. As a statement concerning their physical abilities even that is incorrect as Hobbes himself notes when he claims that even the weakest man can kill the strongest "by confederacy with others."[17] If it takes a group of weak men to kill a strong man this surely is not equality, except insofar as all men are equally mortal, a statement having nothing to do with equal abilities.

With regard to the faculties of the mind, Hobbes is even more clever. He admits that men are vastly unequal in what we may call logical ability. With regard to practical wisdom, Hobbes initially claims it to be distributed equally but then dissolves this assertion into the irrelevant claim that experience bestows its wisdom equally to all those who devote equal time and effort to various pursuits. Finally he suggests that all men seem to believe that their own wit and learning are superior to that of others and concludes with the obviously irrelevant suggestion that "this proveth rather that men are in that point more equal than unequal. For there is not ordinarily a greater sign of the equal distribution of a thing than that every man is contented with his share."[18]

48

Having done with any attempt to prove that human beings are equal in any of these ways, Hobbes proceeds, just as Locke, to assume the equal right of all in the state of nature to preserve themselves with whatever means are at hand. Furthermore, as in Locke's treatment, this discussion ignores the patent disparities among men in both abilities and desires to defend themselves. Men have rights to life which are both equally held and equally inalienable; that is the essence of Hobbes's teaching just as it was of Locke's; both silently admit that such a claim is indemonstrable. Quite the same sort of view of equality as a postulate is found in Rousseau, Kant and many lesser writers.

Rousseau, for example, in *Discourse on the Origin of Inequality*, regards the entry of human beings into society as a cause of inequality. But both *The Social Contract* and *Emile* modify this contention. In *The Social Contract*, equality, in the sense of the equal right to protect oneself from others, is assumed as the basis of the transition from nature to society, precisely as in Hobbes and Locke. In *Emile*, Rousseau shows how the vastly disparate, and hence unequal, passions and capacities of human beings in the state of nature can be tamed and molded in the direction of the equality and sameness which are necessarily found in citizens in democratic regimes.[19] No theorist of the American founding ever seriously disputed this teaching concerning equality. Mostly one finds silent agreement with Jefferson's formulation—it is self-evident, meaning, of course, that it is a necessary but unprovable postulate.[20]

The American Declaration of Independence gives memorable expression of this primeval grounding of the liberal regime; but it was a commonplace in the thought of the statesmen and politicians who brought about the founding of the American regime. In the period of the revolution, many of the American colonies drafted new constitutions which reflected their changed political status. Most of these new constitutions begin with a preamble that acknowledges equality, in the Lockean sense, as the premise of their new enterprise of founding a liberal regime.[21]

One can cite variants of this argument in the writings of

49

most of the founding fathers of the American regime. The core teaching was always equivalent and may be reduced to three essential propositions:

1. human beings are equal in moral standing,
2. the purpose of government is to secure men in the exercise of the rights which they hold equally with their fellows, and
3. consent of the many is necessary because no one is so superior in wisdom that one ought to rule by right.

The regime must treat men as equal in worth, its vision limited to an acknowledgment of an individual's generally similar bodily needs and the natural rights necessary to preserve one's bodily existence. Nothing more was necessary for the founding of just political rule. In fact, the belief that someone actually knew more about human beings, in a politically relevant sense, was regarded as frankly dangerous to the preservation of republican regimes.

Most contemporary liberal theorists either openly or implicitly reach conclusions on the equality principle similar to those found in Hobbes and Locke. They typically admit that there is no specific set of attributes or abilities that all men possess equally, even if it were granted that any such possession were relevant to the question of equal moral standing. Since this cannot be the basis of any version of the equality principle, current theorists conclude that equality, in the sense of equal moral standing or the equal possession of fundamental rights, must be postulated. First, this is done by arguing that to do otherwise runs the risk of undermining the very structure of justice that serves us all tolerably well. This is the route taken by Rawls, who argues for the inclusion of the mentally retarded in the moral community formed by the original contractors on precisely this ground.[22] Secondly, in a related fashion, the notion of equality is said to nurture a "benevolent concern or affection that holds families and communities together." In other words, it nurtures the virtues that make for humane communities of care and concern.[23] Thirdly, there are those who argue that, especially in the matter of fundamental rights, there are no relevant reasons for supposing inequality. This, of course, assumes equality as a norm and then seeks to offer plausible grounds for this assumption; its corollary is that the reasons which might be offered for inequality with respect to fundamental moral standing or rights are either false or irrelevant. The assumption about equality, however, turns out to be just that: an assumption. This point can be seen forcefully in the most persuasive version of the relevant-reasons argument when the author deliberately excludes at a crucial point in the argument people who are mad or mentally defective. To include them requires precisely the postulate that I have been sketching; to exclude them requires giving up the equality principle. [24] Willy-nilly, contemporary theorists offer tacit, if somewhat confusing, testimony to their acceptance of the truth of the position first developed in Locke and Hobbes concerning these matters.

Interpretations of Equality

We have seen that the writings of the founders of liberalism posit equality as an assumed but unproven postulate. This is precisely because the required understanding of equality cannot be demonstrated in any straightforward manner. Though decisive, as we have noted, the belief in human equality is without question the most slippery concept in liberal theory. It is slippery because in many ways it is a dialectical concept. It is, of course, tautologically true that all human beings are equal in as much as they are human: they are equal in their humanity, in their participation in the form of man which enables us to recognize them as human beings. On this level the concept of human equality is essentially empty. But immense problems follow the attempt to put some meaning behind the word *equality*. Basically, it is possible to understand humanity, that in which all human beings equally share, in light either of the high in man's nature, one's powers and capabilities, or of the low, one's basic physiological needs and weaknesses.

In terms of the traditional dichotomy of human nature, humanity can be understood in terms of the body or the soul. But both ways of looking at man render the concept of human

51

equality problematic. On the one hand, it is manifest that human beings are not equal with respect to the soul, in their powers or faculties. The view of human beings as soul leads inevitably to the conviction of human inequality, not equality. Indeed it makes it difficult, if not impossible, to account for the manifest identity, the species relationship of all human beings. It leads to the claim that some individuals are more human than others and perhaps some are not human, or doubtfully human. On the other hand, the view of man as body tends to erase the distinction between the human and the nonhuman and thus to negate the concept of humanity itself and hence the very idea of human equality. Human beings are indeed equal with respect to the needs of the body. In this regard, however, they are qualitatively indistinguishable from nonhuman beings, which also have bodies.

Thus liberalism posits an understanding of human equality that entails two central features. In the first place the essential category, from which the most politically and legally decisive conclusions follow is species membership. Human being is the category of decisive significance, the rest is secondary or frankly dangerous. Members of the species count in liberal theory, entities not members of the species do not, at least not in the same way nor with the same seriousness. Secondly, the worth of each human being, expressed in terms of his possession of equal natural rights which must be respected in political and legal choice, must be assumed. These rights are possessed by every member of the species; no additional qualifications are necessary. To be a member of the species is to bear these rights as a result of nature, that is, they are moral givens. To be a member of the species residing in a given liberal regime is to possess these rights as crucial restrictions on the law and policy of the government. In short, liberal regimes posit the equal worth of all members of the human species as a precondition of those regimes' existence. They stand or fall with the presumption of this understanding of human equality.

But the fact that the conviction of human equality is frequently expressed in terms of individual rights possessed equally by all members of the society must not be miscon-strued. It is true that liberal theory holds to this view of individ-ual rights. But it only expresses in politically useful language a conviction regarding equality that is itself much richer and more fundamental than the belief in individual rights which is grounded on it. This richer understanding of equality is the belief in equal worth or equal dignity which we have already noted. To grasp the significance of such a belief one need only recall that the understanding of individual rights that is part of the constitutive essence of liberal theory is formed by two cen-tral propositions:

1. these rights are special inalienable claims of all human beings, and
2. these rights are possessed especially and only—in this form or with this stringency—by human beings.

The first of these propositions is the one most often seen in the writings of various liberal theorists past and present. Hu-man beings possess special inalienable rights, rights held equally by all human beings. Nevertheless, it still seems evi-dent that unless human beings had some special worth it would make little sense to endow them with the very special moral status which is entailed in the doctrine of natural rights. If it were not presumed that human beings had such worth, there would be no point ascribing to them the special moral status necessarily flowing from the doctrine of natural rights of all human beings. Further if this worth were not possessed by all human beings equally then it would be wrong to view the rights themselves as held equally, as they are indisputably viewed in liberal theory. Such a transformation would entail many impor-tant changes both in the doctrine of natural rights and in the common and statutory law of homicide which clearly views all homicides in various categories—murder, manslaughter, and so forth—with equal seriousness, irrespective of subjective wishes of the victim or his or her qualitative state of life.

To put the point more sharply, the liberal commitment to human freedom, articulated in a doctrine of fundamental rights, requires in its political dimension a belief in equality. Only a belief in the equal worth of every life renders the commitment to political liberty, and hence individual freedom, coherent. If it is proposed that there are ostensibly human beings that do not count as bearers of a right to have their lives protected, then those who know this supposedly know what qualities beyond species membership make life worth living and thus worth protecting. Further, they seem to know this in a politically and jurisprudentially decisive manner. Surely, however, such wisdom ought to be given force in appropriate public policies that would restrict freedom on behalf of whatever virtues do make life worth living and those who possess this knowledge should certainly assume power over those of us less wise in these awesome matters. In fact it would appear that the most unjust thing to do would be to fail to guide the rest of us to this ultimate knowledge through wise restrictions on what we may do with our lives. In this respect the belief in the equal worth of each life and the commitment to liberty stand together.

In this manner equality emerges as the foundation of the political rights of the individual which give structure to the liberty of all. In liberal theory it is because men are equal that they enjoy natural rights; their natural rights flow from and give a measure of substance to their natural equality. In this regard the arrangement in Jefferson's formulation in the "Declaration of Independence" is instructive:

> We hold these truths to be self-evident, that all men are created equal, that they are endowed by their Creator with certain unalienable Rights, that among these are Life, Liberty, and the pursuit of Happiness.

For Jefferson, equality seems to be prior to natural rights. The best way to understand this is to say that it is because men are equal that they enjoy these rights: because all human beings are equal, no one has a superior claim to life, and all have an equal right to life; no one has any right to rule over others, and all have an equal right to liberty; no person is worth more than any other, and all have an equal claim to happiness, or more precisely, an equal right to pursue happiness as they understand it. The liberal abstraction from the concept of a human soul provided the context for the assertion of equality. Human beings are demonstrably not equal except in those characteristics that liberalism made politically decisive—the needs of the body for food, shelter, security and the need for property to stand as a bulwark against anyone who would try to invade the former interests.[25]

Furthermore, we may note that the common and statutory law of most liberal regimes clearly implies a ranking of the importance of various rights which is similar to what one finds in Jefferson's famous formulation. The most serious offenses are those representing a threat to the life of the person. Other offenses are treated with varying degrees of gravity all less severe than those represented by offenses against the life of another person. Again, most classical liberal theorists regarded property rights as extensions of the right to protect oneself from harm. Property was regarded as a necessary bulwark against the hostile forces of the outside world, and as one means whereby a man could supply the material foundations of bodily survival, that is, food and shelter. The primacy of offenses against the person gives expression to the fundamental nature of the premise regarding the equal worth of human beings in liberal theory. The most fundamental way in which such worth could be negated is, of course, the killing of a human being; the common and statutory law of Western liberal regimes regard this as the most serious crime possible.

The primacy of this conviction regarding equality is seen even more clearly in the second of our two propositions, namely, that these rights are possessed only in this fashion by human beings. God has no need of such rights and animals do not merit them, at least with nothing approaching the stringency with which they are possessed by human beings. I do not know of any serious writer who would actually dispute this point in practice. Surely no theologian would claim that God needs inalienable rights to protect him. Insofar as animals are concerned, I still submit that no serious writer would maintain that, if a choice is to be made between killing animals and killing people we should kill people first. This point holds true,

55

I submit, irrespective of the disabilities of human beings involved. If I only have enough food for a starving dog or a starving retarded child, surely the child should not starve before the dog. This is a choice that seems to me basic to the liberal theory of rights and the premises about human worth on which they are based. Human beings count for more than animals.

Once granted, the import of these observations is highly significant. Behind the belief in individual rights and the consent of those ruled to the government that rules them, thus behind liberal government itself, lies the primeval conviction that human beings have an equal worth, or what is more commonly called equality of human dignity. This is the ground whence springs their rights to life and liberty and to a regime capable of sustaining these rights and preventing their alienation. If such a belief is abandoned, it would make little sense to be especially protective of the lives of human beings or to prefer the life and liberty of human beings *per se* to those of various animals. This result would cast doubt on whether a coherent case could be made for liberal government. Little could be said to defend it against the claims of despotic regimes, the likes of which have so blotched political history in the twentieth century. Such a result, of course, is a fundamental departure from the core liberal theory.

In 1790 one of the most important and least read of our founding fathers, James Wilson, the second associate justice of the Supreme Court, wrote:

> When we say that all men are equal we mean not to apply this equality to their talents, dispositions or their acquirements. In all these respects there is and is fit for the great purposes of society that there should be great inequality among men. In the moral and political as well as in the natural world, diversity forms an important part of beauty; and as of beauty, so of utility likewise. That social happiness, which arises from the friendly intercourse of good offices, could not be enjoyed, unless men were so framed and so disposed as mutually to afford and to stand in need of service and assistance. Hence the necessity, not only of great variety but even of great inequality in the talents of

56

men, bodily as well as mental. . . . But however great the
variety and inequality of men may be with regard to virtue,
talent, taste, and acquirements; there is still one aspect in
which all men . . . are equal. With regard to all there is an
equality in rights and obligations; there is that *jus aequum*,
that equal law in which the Romans placed true freedom.
The natural rights and duties of man belong equally to all.
Each forms a part of that great system whose greatest interest and happiness are intended by all the laws of God and
nature. These laws prohibit the wisest and most powerful
from inflicting misery on the meanest and most ignorant;
and from depriving them of their rights or just acquisition.
By these laws, rights natural or acquired are confirmed, in
the same manner to all.[26]

Whether we still accept the belief in divine providence and
natural law which is evident here is doubtful. But Wilson has
articulated the essential understanding of equality and its relation to individual rights on which this regime was founded and
from which we depart only if we are actually prepared to re-
found our polity on a fundamentally different set of organizing
principles.

Viewed in this manner I submit that the public teaching
which underlies liberal political regimes differs fundamentally
from much of the current discussion about the moral significance of persons as distinguished from mere human beings. In
general the argument is that some set of characteristics, beyond
those of species membership, distinguishes a human being
from a person. These characteristics are either necessary or
sufficient conditions for intrinsically valuing persons and viewing them as bearers of fundamental moral rights, such as a right
to life. Only persons are intrinsically valuable and ought to be
regarded in law and policy as the possessors of fundamental
rights that set limits on how they may be treated.[27]

To view these characteristics as sufficient to lead to the
desired conclusion would be to derive a moral conclusion about
rights and value from a set of supposed facts, a move that does
not find favor in current moral philosophy. The more typical
move is to regard these characteristics of persons as necessary

conditions for the ascription of rights to the individual and corresponding duties to others. The result is that taking the life of a nonperson or mere human being is much less serious than the murder of a person; often, it may not be morally wrong at all. Surely, abortion or infanticide in the typical case of conception by impoverished mothers or the birth of a severely handicapped infant would be plainly acceptable since neither the fetus nor the neonate could properly be said to be a person with intrinsic rights or worth.

Of course, the precise characteristics that are necessary for persons are a matter of dispute but it is generally acknowledged that they must be psychological capacities, not physical attributes. That is, it must be some set of mental attributes that require a certain level of neurological development and psychological awareness as their basis. The most common move at this point is to focus as Michael Tooley does on intellectual capacities such as "being capable of having desires" or being "an enduring subject of nonmomentary interests" or possessing consciousness of oneself as a "continuing subject of mental experiences."[28] Whatever the precise formulation it seems doubtful that any such formulation can be given that will be satisfactory to the advocates of this position. Consider, for example, the view that the capacity for desires or interests is the crucial characteristic of the person. If desires or interests or other "thought episodes" are viewed as essentially propositional, requiring linguistic capacities of the person we have clearly gone too far for no good reason. At the very least such capacities are not just missing from the fetus and the neonate. Literally hundreds of thousands of profoundly and severely retarded or senile persons may lack any of these linguistic capacities. As such, on this account they would not be persons with fundamental rights. On the other hand, once we give up the notion that thought episodes are propositional in form it seems doubtful that anyone would be excluded from being a person: the usefulness of the person–human being distinction would be negligible. If we regard interests or desires as present simply when there is a repeated avoidance of painful or otherwise aversive conditions, it seems that doubtful that any human being is excluded . As we shall see in chapter five, response to ostensibly painful stimuli begins to occur at least as early as the second half of the first trimester of pregnancy, just when the gross anatomical and physiological features of the species are also complete in the fetus. Surely this seems not what was originally intended by the "human–person" distinction.

In other words, if we conclude that to be "continuing subject of mental experiences" one must have the mental capacity to express experiences in propositional form then we have surely gone to far and we have excluded all those who cannot let us know that they have the requisite abilities. On the other hand, if we conclude that to be a person with interests one only has to manifest the behavioral responses consistent with having certain sorts of experiences, which certainly seems to better reflect our common means of interpersonal knowledge, then the distinction originally sought seems to evaporate.[29]

The most fundamental weakness in the view that attaches significance to the distinction between human beings and persons is the notion that the liberal theory of rights is derived from essentially metaphysical premises about person. On such a view, claims about individual political rights are at least partially justified by claims about the nature of human persons. If this approach to rights is accepted, it makes sense to ask what the nature of persons is and what it is that makes them intrinsically valuable or "endowed" with "inalienable rights."[30]

Once this move is made, we are bound to find that the range of human ability is so great that we cannot possibly find abilities beyond the most minimal that are held equally by everyone. In short we are bound to come to an inegalitarian notion of rights, such as embodied in the current discussion of rights and persons. Liberal political philosophy, however, is simply not prepared to ask any of these questions. In other words, the very idea that rights are based on some metaphysical attributes of person is foreign to liberalism, for the liberal theory of rights is a social practice, a postulate of political order if you will, that is deliberately set forth because of a profound skepticism about metaphysical and moral knowledge of the sort that is under discussion here. The antimetaphysical bias of the founders of classical liberalism is well known. Their political philosophy is drenched in it. Likewise, their moral teaching displays none of the certainties about the human good that are found in Aquinas or Hooker. Even when Locke tells us that with proper effort morality can be made as certain as mathematics, the moral truths he actually produces are only of the simple, didactic sort that one finds in the decalogue.

Unlike the recent discussion of persons, the classical liberals drew their greatest inspiration and firmest grounding not from metaphysics but from history. In Hobbes, for example, it was the dismal record of metaphysical politics in his own time, that is, the Puritan revolution, that gave force to his skeptical claims about the mixing of metaphysics and politics. For Hume it is likewise his mammoth *History of England* that provides the crucial link between his radically skeptical philosophy and his extremely conservative politics. History supposedly demonstrated the practical wisdom of liberal political regimes, divorced from the metaphysical and moral theorizing that guided ancient and medieval political philosophy. These are precisely the same sorts of theorizing that animate the current discussion about the moral significance of person which likewise cannot form the basis of stable humane community life.

Inalienability of Human Rights

From the equal possession of natural rights, both Hobbes and Locke derive the justness of liberal government. The equality of men means that no man is so superior in wisdom or virtue that he ought to rule as a matter of right, nor is one so superior in one's standing that one can justly demand the abrogation or alienation of individual rights, as God is said in some theological systems to be able to do. Since no one person has a true right to rule each has an equal right to rule, insofar as justice is concerned. But no regime could, of course, be founded on this basis for both practical and theoretical reasons. Hence Hobbes and Locke found government on a popular basis: the consent of the governed and the transfer of actual governmental power to those few by whom the many consent to be governed.[31]

Moreover, any such just government must be limited in

principle by the necessity of respecting the inalienable rights of the individual. The claim that inalienable rights exist is much disputed in contemporary thought; yet they are an indispensable part of the heritage of liberal regimes. On such rights the founders of classical liberalism held two crucial propositions.

First, they held that in some situations a regime cannot protect all inalienable rights equally. Such was the case with war. In war the soldier is properly called to protect both his and his fellow citizen's rights out of the belief that the alternative is worse: the loss of everyone's rights, including the soldier's, by subjugation to a foreign tyranny. This of course is a difficult matter to judge correctly and it is one of the reasons that foreign affairs and defense matters are the most complex and difficult questions which statesmen of whatever political persuasion face. Granting it, however, does not materially alter the truth of the idea of inalienable rights. It merely testifies to the imperfections of human existence, the very imperfections which, in liberal theory, make political rule necessary and the doctrines of rights and limited government indispensable to just political rule. It remains true that, for the founders of classical liberalism, government must respect inalienable rights without the extreme case where it cannot do so equally and must send some to war to preserve the rights of the many.[32]

Secondly, the founders held that inalienable rights could not justly be alienated by anyone, even by the individual himself. To hold otherwise would be to give up the notion entirely and hence the notion of limited popular government. Here Hobbes was blunt: a man who seemed to give up his right to self-preservation and release his fellows from their corresponding obligations simply did not know what he was doing. "He is not to be understood as if he meant it or that it was his will, but that he was ignorant of how such words and actions are to be interpreted."[33] The moves by which Hobbes and Locke are led to this conclusion are crucial for understanding liberal government. Both Hobbes and Locke wanted to deny the justness of tyrannical regimes that would enslave their citizens in various ways either overtly or covertly. However, in rejecting classical political philosophy, they foreclose its answer to the enslaving tyrant's claim to rule, namely, that the tyrant departs from the rule of justice itself in the direction of self-interest. The subject is, of course, more complex than this; the tyrant does not always have no claim to rule since the alternative may be worse— anarchy of the worst sort. But in general, classical political philosophy saw tyranny as unjust in principle precisely because the tyrant departed from the rule of justice in the direction of self-aggrandizement.[34] The alternative response in Hobbes and Locke is found in the doctrine of inalienable rights, which provide the limit to governmental authority and the answer to the claims of those who would seek to go beyond those limits. However, if one could alienate one's most fundamental right, the right to life, one surely could justly alienate any lesser right such as liberty. In short, one could justly sell oneself into slavery or, what is the same thing, consent to a government that had absolute power over him.[35] Given the necessity of relying on assumed or tacit consent in most cases of governmental action, it becomes an impossible matter to judge which governments have proper consent of the governed without the belief in rights which government must respect to be just and therefore merit the consent of the governed. Without such a premise, despotic regimes that enslave or execute their citizens at will would become just merely on their own say-so. Both Hobbes and especially Locke want to maintain the view that there are inherent limits to what government may justly demand of its citizens. To do this requires a limit to both what government may justly demand from the individual and what rights the individual may alienate.

On both of these points, liberal, free government stands or falls on the premise of equally held and inalienable rights of individuals. Deny the equal and special rights of individuals in this regard and one denies both the correctness of popular consent to government and the justness of limits on the power of the government over its citizens. Government then might be just if it acted with no overt consent from its citizens and in complete defiance of individual rights. To deny that any such result could be in accord with justice and to establish the justice of the liberal alternative is the essential burden of the teaching of Hobbes and Locke on the essence and essential interconnections of equality, inalienable rights, and liberal government.

The commitment of liberal regimes to equality about the most minimal rights of individuals stemmed in the first instance from an overt rejection of the political philosophy of the ancients. In a curious way, however, the ancients may remain our best teachers. At one level the whole meaning of Plato's *Republic* is precisely what liberal theorists have always maintained. The *Republic* is a regime in speech, which, like the vision of the good, dialectically illuminates the enterprise of political rule in ordinary regimes. Still it is a regime in speech, not in practice. As such, it demonstrates what would be required to make such a regime ruled by the perfectly wise and just a reality. For our purposes we note one essential feature, namely, the absence of a written law that might restrain the activities of the ruler. In essence, Plate and Aristotle taught that it is impossible to capture in written law the judgments necessarily entailed in the establishment and governance of a regime like that of the *Republic*. Aside from the obvious points made in this regard in the *Republic, Laws,* and *Statesman,* the most telling example of Plato's teaching is dialectic between the *Apology,* where Socrates knows that injustice is being done, and the *Crito,* where he nevertheless obeys the law. As the *Republic* makes clear, law cannot account for the extraordinary man such as Socrates.

With the ancients, the founders of liberalism understood that, in actual societies, wisdom does not rule and hence justice is not to be found in the unrestrained rule of those who govern. They had too many memories of absolute power abused and they knew too much history to be very sanguine concerning the virtues of those who attain positions of political power.

In fact, this very point appears as one of the central teachings of Plato's other dialogue, the *Laws.* Consider, for example, the teaching on infanticide, a matter of special concern to us in this book. Plato's endorsement of selective infanticide for defective infants occurs only in the *Republic.*[36] Need we be reminded that this regime is ruled over by those whose perfect wisdom would surely encompass a knowledge of when it might be just to conclude that some members of the species do not even merit the most minimal protections that any regime can provide to its citizens. In the *Laws*, however, a regime ruled by rather ordinary aging politicians, the law on homicide, especially homicide of one's children, is fundamentally different.[37] This difference points to the essential problem of deciding when some members of the species do not count in a politically or legally decisive sense. Only in a regime like that of the *Republic*, where perfect wisdom rules, can such ultimate justice be safely allowed to operate. Like Plato, the founders of modern liberal regimes knew that such wisdom simply does not exist among ordinary mortals and that, even if some few possess it, they have little chance of gaining or holding positions of political rule.

Liberal Regimes as Rule of Law

Since unrestrained rule inevitably degenerated into a tyranny of the one or the many, the only possible political regimes with even a semblance of justice were those that based themselves on written law. "Law," Blackstone observed, "is a rule; not a transient or sudden order from a superior to or concerning a particular person; but something permanent, uniform, universal."[38] In this sense, written law and constitutions served to codify the minimum rights and responsibilities of the people against the inevitable tendency toward one of the many forms of tyranny in political life.[39] Of course, the rule of law is also found in various versions in classic and medieval thought. In medieval times these versions are all rooted in the Stoic *logos* doctrine. The fundamental difference between the medieval view of the rule of law and characteristically modern, liberal views is the medieval insistence on human reason as a necessary ingredient in understanding the logos in nature. This means that political prudence stood outside the rule of written positive law, and could itself reach just decisions through an immediate grasp of the natural law as *logos*. In modern times political prudence is distrusted and therefore those who rule are themselves said to be constrained by written positive laws and constitutions.[40]

Liberal regimes are thus preeminently regimes of the rule of law. This follows in two senses. Having rejected the natural sociability of man, modern political thought replaces it with a set of legal conventions that become the bonds which hold society together. To be without law is to be without government, reduced to the animal status described in the many versions of the state of nature that is an endemic part of liberal theory. "Government without laws," writes Locke, "is, I suppose, a mystery in politics, inconceivable to human capacity and inconsistent with human society."[41]

The liberal commitment to the rule of law, however, meant more than this notion of social bonds. As Locke notes in the context of the above sentence, there is an intimate connection between the rule of law and the securing of liberal justice, that is, securing men in the exercise of their rights. Written law provides a general framework that transcends the passions of the many and the fleeting judgment of the few. The rule of law assures equality about basic rights by ignoring the claims of those who assert themselves as being so superior in virtue or knowledge that they can act against another's rights with just impunity. In rejecting the claims of such individuals, liberal regimes posit the superiority of law and thus reaffirm their commitment to equality by denying a place to those who would destroy both either by their claims to superiority or outrageous behavior. Thus, liberal regimes codify in law the fundamental rights held equally by all citizens, that is, by all human beings governed by the regime. This is the maneuver which translates the conviction regarding the equal worth of each human being into legally and politically relevant terms. All human beings have these rights to which civil law gives effect and in the shadow of which public policy must be formed.

In this regard liberalism shows a profound distrust of discretionary authority to bend legal rules to fit the shape of specific cases or to disregard them altogether in the pursuit of justice in a particular instance. The founders of liberalism, especially

65

those engaged in the establishment of actual political regimes, deeply suspected such authority, especially as it regarded domestic affairs that directly impinged on the rights of citizens.[42]

Lacking a knowledge of perfect justice and believing such knowledge both exceedingly rare and politically impotent, the founders of liberalism knew that such discretionary authority is all too often a mask for the gravest injustices. Without the wisdom of Socrates or Solomon, one man's discretionary justice is another's tyranny. Liberalism, we must remember, deliberately presented itself as a regime based on and tailored to the demands of human imperfection. Such imperfection would almost inevitably distort discretionary power for evil purposes or would produce such disparities of treatment as to render the result patently unjust.

That the framers were correct in these assumptions is, I believe, obvious when one examines even cursorily the areas of domestic policy touching on fundamental rights, where discretion is given very substantial room to maneuver. Consider just the two processes of granting bail and criminal sentencing. In both cases it was originally believed that allowing a wide latitude for judicial discretion would provide for remedies tailored to the case at hand, thus producing a substantially more just result than the alternatives.[43] But what have resulted are gross disparities in the treatment of demonstrably similar suspects or convicted offenders and the loss of even the semblance of minimally adequate fairness. Currently many responsible spokesmen across the political spectrum are calling for the imposition of fixed minimum sentences for offenders and for either the elimination or sharp curtailment of the bail system. One can document similar patterns of injustices in other areas where powerful discretionary authority prevails, such as a prosecutor's decision to prosecute,[44] or a police officer's discretion to say that a crime has occurred and invoke the criminal justice system in response.[45]

Of course, none of this means that there are no exceptions to legal rules or that public policies cannot be sufficiently nuanced to take account of the complexities of civic life. What it does mean is that exceptions to legal rules, especially as they

66

affect fundamental rights, must be stated in such a manner that they do not render the rule impotent or its enforcement impossible. They must be clear, coherent, and generalizable, neither intrinsically bound to the particularities of special cases nor providing the basis for everyone to become the judge of one's own case and thereby escape the application of the rule by appealing to something unique to oneself such as feelings or desires. To be acceptable, an exception to a rule must not destroy the force of the general rule itself.

As an example of this problem, consider two sorts of cases. First consider self-defense exceptions to a homicide law. These exceptions are generally capable of fairly precise delineation in terms independent of the particularities of the specific case at hand. There are, of course, wide divergences among American jurisdictions concerning when a self-defense exception may be invoked but in each jurisdiction the exception itself can usually be framed and applied so that the general rule against homicide is not rendered impotent. A second sort of case is the legal rule against assisting in suicide. The rule has no exceptions because it appears impossible to formulate any which would not destroy the force of the general rule. Even the most ardent defenders of the right to commit suicide and to assist others in committing suicide only claim it is justified in a few cases. Therefore, exceptions to the legal rule regarding assisting in suicide would need to be framed so as to distinguish justified acts from what is normally regarded as the most serious of moral and legal wrongs, homicide or assisting in homicide. As we shall see in another chapter, none of those who seek to offer legal protection to those who assist in the commission of suicide have produced even modestly persuasive drafts of possible exception clauses.[46] Even granting that such a clause could be produced, there would remain a serious objection to an exception clause which would render enforcement of the rule itself difficult if not impossible when the victim and very possibly the only witness is now dead. Hence even if we grant the theoretical possibility of justifiable exceptions to the rule, the rule itself remains because of the impossibility of formulating any of those exceptions in an acceptable manner.[47]

Finally, we note that the liberal understanding of human equality does not mean that all human beings are similar in their desires or equal in mental or moral capacities. Such differences are obvious facts of human existence and no one would wish to ignore them. Neither does this understanding of equality imply anything concerning the just distribution of material goods and services. Perhaps a given distribution of wealth is unjust. If it is, the case made for such a claim cannot be deduced from the liberal premise of the worth of each human life.

Slavery: Critical Case for Nineteenth Century Liberalism

In the American political experience, the most penetrating articulation of this understanding of the liberal, especially the American, regime comes from Abraham Lincoln. The issue that Lincoln confronted, slavery, posed a fundamental challenge to a regime based on equality and liberty. As such it was necessary for Lincoln to confront the central questions regarding the core of liberal government in his attempt to understand the evil of slavery and the remedies that might be applied to bring about its end. With great insight Lincoln penetrated to the core of the problem and laid bare the challenge of slavery in manner that is powerfully relevant to the contemporary issues we are dealing with here. Slavery, of course, was part of the constitution, but, as Lincoln well knew, that was more the result of the politcal realities of 1787 than a well-thought-out rationale in the mind of the founders. With slavery already in existence, it simply had to be given some status, or the whole constitutional enterprise would never have succeeded.[48]

But slavery itself was incompatible in the long run with the principle of civil equality on which liberal government stands or falls. That, in essence, was the overt message that Lincoln carried to his audiences in the troubled years before the Civil War. The two, he argued, cannot coexist indefinitely. One principle will destroy the other. If Congress was to be empowered to make it lawful for one man to enslave another, then this principle itself could logically be extended *ad infinitum*. Slavery would eventually destroy freedom by turning it from a right enjoyed by all to a privilege enjoyed by the majority.[49]

The deeper impulse behind Lincoln's belief in the incompatibility of slavery and the American regime is seen only obliquely in his speeches but the meaning is undeniable. Slavery does not just treat one man as better than another or as entitled to privileges that another may not enjoy. Lincoln himself was quite comfortable with such divisions among human abilities and a system of merit rewards based on them. Rather, the fundamental evil in slavery was that it treated one ostensible human being as if he or she were not a human being at all, insofar as political status was concerned. More than denying that the enslaved person had all the rights and privileges of another, slavery ended up asserting that the enslaved had no rights at all. In political terms the enslaved was no longer a human being entitled to the inalienable rights with which all men are supposedly endowed.[50]

The black human being was thus dehumanized not in some abstract sense but in the most primeval sense of all. He or she was summarily counted out of the human family for political purposes. He or she was now a "brute" in Lincoln's word, no longer even human. This was the most fundamental evil of slavery: it denied the moral and political status of the slave as one whose life and freedom should be protected by the American regime. The slave not only had no freedom; he or she further had no moral status from which to claim liberty and to seek from the community the minimal protections due to other ostensibly human individuals. The fundamental evil of slavery was thus its denial of the equal human standing of the slave, which is the necessary premise of the assertion of one's right to a liberty fit for human beings as opposed to a slavery fit for animals.

Lincoln knew full well that this view of the status of blacks was fundamentally inconsistent with the charter of American government—the *Declaration of Independence*. The point he drove home with relentless force was simply that a liberal regime, dedicated to the principles of freedom and basic equality, could not consistently decide to treat some human beings as not even possessed of the most minimal political rights. In one of his most significant speeches, at Columbus, Ohio, in September 1859, he put his argument in its most succinct form:

> I ask attention to the fact that to a preeminent degree these popular sovereigns are at this work: blowing out the moral lights around us. Teaching that the negro is no longer a man but a brute, that the Declaration has nothing to do with him, that he ranks with the crocodile and the reptile, that a man with body and soul is a matter of dollars and cents. I suggest to this portion of Ohio Republicans, or Democrats, if there be any present, the serious consideration of this fact that there is now going on among you a steady process of debauching public opinion on this subject.[51]

The reference to "popular sovereigns" in the above passage suggests Lincoln's most far-reaching point. His great opponent, Douglas, had stood on the principle of popular sovereignty which translated to the proposition that if the people of a given territory wanted slavery they should be allowed to have it.[52] At its face value this seemed like the perfect embodiment of the essential principles of liberal government—the absoluted sovereignty of popular will expressed by the majority of citizens. For Lincoln this deceptively simple proposition was nothing less than an insidious assault on the possibility of liberal democratic government. Lincoln knew better than his opponents that liberal governments survive only because the principles on which they are based are themselves not open to question in the same manner as the many other questions of public policy with which the majority may rightly concern itself. Liberalism as a set of principles embodied in a particular regime must transcend the matrix of free decision making that it protects. Without this, liberty turns on itself and ends up destroying the very freedom employed in the first place. As Professor Jaffa has pungently remarked, "Douglas insisted upon the rights of communities to manage their domestic affairs in the same way that Lincoln insisted upon the inalienable rights of man."[53]

In Douglas's view popular sovereignty amounted to the proposition that the majority of the people could rightfully decide to repeal the fundamental charter of the American regime. For Lincoln this was the ultimate perversion of democratic government: the regime allowed its own systematic destruction, not by overtly permitting the corruption of public sentiment but by allowing the insidious notion of popular sovereignty to spread out unchallenged. As evil as it was, slavery was hardly comparable to this covert destruction of a regime which, given time, would uproot slavery from its midst.

Worthlessness of Some Human Lives: Critical Case for Modern Liberalism

Lincoln's articulation of the core of the liberal—the American—political teaching and its relation to the slavery question leads us to the heart of the discussion in this book. Slavery could not be permitted as a matter of law and public policy, irrespective of whatever utilitarian or other moral case might be made for it. It was unjust because it denied the very basis of the regime itself. As such, one would have to give: either the regime remained what it was and legally protected slavery was banished in time, or the regime itself would be fundamentally altered in making a permanent commitment to its presence.

But slavery is only one way in which the equal worth of human beings can be denied in public policy and law. Men can certainly treat other men as animals without enslaving them overtly as the horrible examples of national socialist, fascist and Stalinist regimes of recent memory and contemporary practice attest. In all of these instances, the essential challenge to liberal theory is the same: some human beings are not believed to merit the minimum protection that a regime can provide equally to all of its citizens. They have lives that simply should not be protected in a politically or legally decisive sense either because of their skin color, their religion, their ethnic heritage, their mental infirmities, or their physical handicaps. Some human beings have lives that are worth protecting and in that sense they have rights to such protection; other human lives simply

71

are not worth living and have no such right to protection. The core issue is as simple and disturbing as that.

Unfortunately, this sort of belief is not limited to the evil regimes of the past or the totalitarian societies of the present. The proposition regarding the worthlessness of some human lives is pressed with increasing vigor on several fronts in Western liberal regimes. The specifics of these arguments will be discussed in the different contexts in which they arise in the following chapters. Here I wish to raise the more general and most fundamental point, namely, that these writers ask us to enact into law and public policy a wholesale departure from the premises of the regime itself. We are being asked to state in law and policy that some lives are not worth living anymore and that someone—physician, family member, friend, caretaker, or court—may decide when this is the case and then take the awesome steps one is normally forbidden to take and cause the death of a human being.

Let us look at an example. If a parent has a sick child, he or she must provide the care necessary to meet the basic needs of the child, especially the care necessary to protect the life of the child. If one fails to do so and the child dies, one is legally liable for prosecution under neglect statutes. Even a claim of fidelity to religious belief will not prevent prosecution and punishment. The law at this point offers equal protection to each child because his or her life has worth irrespective of the desires or beliefs of the parents or the handicaps that burden his or her existence. This principle is embodied in a hundred years of Anglo-American case law, in which courts almost routinely order life-saving therapy for children over the objections of parents.[54] But now we are being told that the law ought to remove its protective shield for some children. In other words, the parents ought to be permitted to act in ways normally held to be serious violations of the criminal neglect statutes solely because they or their physicians believe that the life of the child is not worth living. In short, the child has too many handicaps, too much retardation, too much bowel incontinence, or too much of some other disability to qualify for the protection of the law in the most minimal manner.

72

This argument is being pressed on us in several different ways in different cases. We will later treat their specifics. The claim is always the same. Some people do not count as other people. They can be treated as if they did not have the rights that others have. If we have made any point at all in the earlier portions of this chapter, it is that such a policy represents a momentous departure from the organizing principles of a liberal regime. To adopt such a policy is not merely to ask for a change in one or another isolated law or public policy. It is to ask that we change the constitutive premises of the regime, those coeval with its existence. Essentially the claim is now being made that someone does know what gives human life its worth, beyond the physiological basis of species membership. Whatever this is, it is something not held equally by all. Some members of the species possess so little of it that they merit no social protection at all. Something beyond mere species membership is the basis of individual rights and the corresponding legal rules and social conventions that oblige others to respect these rights. Those who have this elusive quality count in a sense decisive for public policy; those who lack it should not count. That is the deceptively simple and troubling position that now begs our acceptance.

Conclusion

Ironically, the case made for this policy, in all of its variations, turns out to be the best possible example of the wisdom of the beliefs that define the existence of liberal regimes. As we shall see throughout the rest of this book, no one who defends the proposition that some lives are not worth living can tell us anything meaningful or plausible about precisely what this quality is, or more important, exactly how much of it one needs to qualify as a possessor of individual rights and the attendant social protections. What they do tell us is sometimes self-contradictory, usually dangerously elastic in its policy implications when fairly applied, and often seriously at odds with other writers who favor some other quality or threshold for the granting of rights and protections.

73

Of course, this was precisely the point of the founders of liberalism when they broke with the classical tradition. No one knows the ultimate answer to these sorts of questions and those who do are simply pretenders to the throne of wisdom. The few who really might know, like Plato's Socrates, will be wise enough to be silent. They will know that a little such knowledge in the hands of the unschooled masses and the powerful few breeds the worst of evils. Even a cursory examination of the numerous attempts to state when life is not worth living will reveal the profound truth of the premises of liberal regimes and, as we shall see, our hapless exile from civilization and humanity when we desert them.

CHAPTER THREE

Infanticide

Introduction

For centuries the most serious obligations of the Western moral and political tradition have been those involving the family. The obligation of parents to provide adequate care for their children and the reciprocal obligations of children toward their parents are among those which moralists of every age and of widely differing theoretical persuasions have stressed with vigor and precision. The parental obligation to the child was likewise clearly articulated in the common law and is now firmly entrenched in the laws of every Western nation and every American state code. Though the penalties for failure to provide adequate care differ, the principle that the child is to be cared for irrespective of his or her lot in life or the lot of the family, is firmly rooted in our moral tradition, public ethos, and our laws and policies.[1]

It is true that these moral and legal presumptions did not prevent the practice of infanticide, especially in Western Europe. Some historians have suggested that this practice was the chief means of population control in Western Europe from the end of the Middle Ages down to the nineteenth century.[2] Even in Victorian England deliberate infanticide was not unknown.[3] The evidence is clear that it was widespread; how much so is a matter of dispute. It was especially prevalent among unmarried women who faced not only the burden of caring for an infant in squalid circumstances but the crushing stigma of unwed motherhood as well.

Despite the pervasiveness of the practice, it was condemned almost universally by moralists, jurists, and criminologists alike. The law consistently refused to countenance it, even if it did act with leniency toward those charged with the practice. This leniency does not, I believe, indicate lesser concern for the life of the infant but results from the special circumstances in which most such offenses occurred, circumstances which made prosecution for homicide almost impossible.

In a detailed historical survey, Catherine Damme intends to demonstrate that, at law, infanticide has always constituted a special case of homicide, not simply another instance of it. Hence, she argues, the newborn has not been treated as a person in this respect in Anglo-American law. To reach this conclusion, she is forced to set aside most of the formal statutory enactments which define the act as murder—such as *Bracton*—and examine societal and legal responses to actual cases, which were broad and lenient. But here the evidence misses the point. As an example, if legal retribution were slight, she concludes that an infant was not valued as much as an adult life. But, in the seventeenth century, women who committed infanticide were considered insane precisely because the act was seen as so heinous that no rational person would do it. She takes the finding of insanity as evidence of leniency. This is done in the face of contemporary records attesting plainly to the special hatred with which the act was viewed.

Furthermore, she discounts completely the connection between the leniency of punishment and the offense with which a person could, in fact be charged. The most common form of child murder was overlaying, in which the infant could be smothered by the mother sleeping on it. But in the conditions of the time, this was also a common form of accidental death. Distinguishing culpability in such cases would be almost impossible; a charge of homicide could rarely be proven. At most, one of the lesser degrees of manslaughter or negligent death might be sustained, but these offenses have always had much lesser penalties attached.[4]

Even the great humanists of the Enlightenment, who sternly critiqued the social and legal attitudes toward unwed motherhood which often led to infanticide, gave little support for the practice itself. However much they sympathized with the plight of the woman, they abhorred her deed.[5]

This consensus of reasoned opinion no longer exists. In the last decade one finds an increasing number of philosophers, physicians, legal scholars, and religious moralists defending courses of action that would knowingly entail the death of some infants born with serious physical or mental handicaps. Some writers have argued frankly for the active killing of supposedly defective infants.[6] Most, however, have only argued that for some infants it would be proper to withdraw or withhold care designed to save their lives yet unable to cure the disabilities which the children would be forced to live with. Substantial advances in neonatal medicine have enabled physicians to save or sustain the lives of increasing numbers of severely disabled infants. As the abilities of physicians have increased in this regard so too has the discussion of the moral and policy issues surrounding the use of these measures. Stirred by what they see as the burden of severe disabilities many writers have opted for abandoning these children to the lethal progress of their ailments, much as an unwed mother of two centuries ago may have abandoned her bastard to the not so tender mercy of the street, in full knowledge that the child would die without care.[7]

The discussion surrounding the termination of the lives of defective newborns may be the most voluminous of any of those that we shall discuss here. Despite much commentary, most of it supporting either active or passive infanticide, the argument I am making in this book is nowhere better displayed. The vagueness and incoherence of claims about the quality of these lives becomes clear on the inspection of such claims in this literature. The logical expansiveness of such claims to cover hundreds of thousands of retarded, disabled, or mentally ill individuals also becomes increasingly clear. The criteria offered to provide answers to these queries are themselves extraordinarily imprecise and confused; sometimes they lead to strongly counterintuitive claims that few would support openly. In short, the departure from the organizing principles of liberal regimes is so marked and the actual policy proposals so confused, so logically expansive, and so unfair in operation that one questions why this discussion has proceeded at this level for so long. But before we can see the weakness of the case being made for selective infanticide, we must be clear just what this case is.

Though some of the medical details may be slightly outdated, the essential case for the selective nontreatment of some newborn infants was stated with great clarity by a leading physician more than a decade and a half ago:

> In our clinic it is not customary to operate on newborn infants or those in the first few months of life with thoracolumbar or upper lumbar myelomeningoceles or myeloschises who exhibit complete sphincter paraplegia below the upper lumbar segments. This is true whether or not there is significant hydrocephalus at the time. When examination in the first day of life, therefore, confirms the total absence of neurologic function below the upper lumbar levels custodial care only is recommended. It is recognized that some of these totally paralyzed hydrocephalic patients recommended for custodial care survive for considerable periods of time. For these patients and their families, it is the doctor's and the community's responsibility to provide this care and to minimize suffering; but at the same time it is also their responsibility not to prolong such individual, familial and community suffering unnecessarily and not to carry out multiple procedures and prolonged expensive acute hospitalization in an infant whose chance for acceptable growth and development is negligible.[8]

As seen in this passage, the case for the selective termination of some newborn lives involves two sets of concerns. First are those relating to the suffering of the family caring for the infant. The second relate to the plight of the infant itself. While these are often joined together in the literature, clearly the second consideration is primary. It is only because the infant is suffering that the burden on the family may be thought to justify not providing life-saving medical therapy. As a practical matter, most parents will not suffer unbearably unless the infant is severely handicapped.

This point can be made in a more telling fashion if we consider a severely physically handicapped adolescent, who may yet have strong mental abilities that could enable him or her to be productive or even brilliant in later life. Surely, the suffering of the family caring for such a person provides no reason for terminating his or her life by withholding medical care the next time it is needed. Consider also an unusual case in which parents suffered greatly with a newborn child who was nevertheless normal in his or her potential. Would the burdens of such a family provide any reason to withhold medical care the next time this infant needed it? Clearly the answer is no. This is the plain import of at least a century of common and statutory law development in which the parent is regarded as having no right to withhold life-saving medical care for a child for any reason.

It therefore conclusively appears that any policy of selective termination or medical neglect of infants' lives will entail selection criteria that focus on the condition of the child and only secondarily, and considering the defects of the child, on the plight of the family and the burdens borne by the society. Seen in this light any selection criteria for distinguishing those infants from whom care can be withheld will involve a judgment that an infant with certain handicaps has a life not worth living. Some authors that we will discuss fail to heed the demands of this requirement. But insofar as they do ignore its implications, their proposals lapse into policies that create the worst sorts of injustices. It is clear on inspection, therefore, that the structure of the argument for the selective termination of the lives of some children brings us back to the essential proposition of Englehardt: sometimes the continued existence of an infant is an injury to that infant. In such a case life itself is a harm and death is preferable.[9] If the first duty of the parents and the physicians is to avoid harm to the child, then the termination of such a life is perfectly compatible with that duty.

Claims about the burden of life to the infant are quite confusing. Usually they seem to represent nothing more than the biases of the authors involved. Consider, in this regard, a recent essay by Richard Brandt in which he proposes that we establish a happiness curve for individual infants centered around an "indifference axis." The curve would go above the line for a moment of happiness and below it for a moment of unhappiness. On the basis of such a curve, he believes, we could decide when some lives are "bad on the whole." Brandt advises the active killing of such infants. Typically, he never gives us any clear idea of how we could decide where to place any given moment on the curve.[10]

Even prescinding from the lack of criteria, the proposal is contradictory on its face. Brandt argues that the neonate has no wants, desires, or experiences that are the basis for the exercise of consent. The child cannot care about life since he or she knows nothing of it. Grant this and the judgment of his "happiness curve" becomes the worst example of arbitrary paternalism. We decide not that one will think one's life bad—we cannot know what the child will think—but rather, that we believe the life will be bad. Why? Simply because we would not want it ourselves? No other alternative seems to exist on Brandt's own ground. For example, he writes: "There are also some positive enjoyments: of eating, drinking, elimination, seeing the nurse coming with food and so on. But those brief enjoyments can hardly balance the long stretches of boredom, discomfort or even pain. On the whole, the lives of such children are bad according to the happiness criterion."[11] Severely abnormal children are hardly ever in pain for long periods so as a description of those he wishes to kill this will not do. Discomfort and boredom are no better. Brandt surely finds boredom unpleasant and believes that the life of the defective child will be boring for long periods. Boring for Brandt, yes. Boring for the child, probably not. At the very least, on Brandt's own grounds we have no way to say whether the infant's life will be boring; to assert that it is only betrays a prejudice against severely abnormal infants and children. In the end Brandt gives us little more than a circle in which to find the answers that are missing from his essay. The lives in question are bad because he asserts that they are bad.

Not only are these claims about the lives of defective newborn children arbitrary; they also lead to strongly counterintuitive results. Severely retarded persons rarely live in pain for long periods. Therefore, the argument for selective death for some newborns must rest not on pain *per se* but on the suffering of these children as they grow. But suffering is a relative phenomenon. Those at the lowest end of the scale of cognitive abilities and social skills do not usually suffer very much. They are little aware of the lives they could be leading were they not afflicted with the handicaps they bear. This knowledge, which is the source of suffering, increases as the degree of handicap diminishes. Therefore, Lorber is right when he notes that, among those children afflicted with spina bifida, the worst off in terms of suffering are those who are mentally normal but physically very handicapped.[12] Therefore Brandt should conclude that those infants whose mental disabilities are only moderate and mild will be those who should have necessary medical care withheld. This conclusion contradicts much of what has been written on the subject but it seems to me that it follows from the premises of Brandt's argument.

Furthermore, those who approach the IQ norm have the best chance of leading worthwhile lives and being productive citizens. These are the people who can benefit from special education and training programs, from group homes, from sheltered workshops, and from psychological counseling. Those who favor the termination of some of these lives must then believe that death is preferable to the expense and effort involved in offering the proper sorts of help and counseling from which these children might benefit. Such a conclusion is both utterly counterintuitive and in contradiction to the public policies and community ethos of every country in the Western world. An argument that leads to these sorts of results is, I believe, untenable at the outset.

Criteria for Selection

These problems are only preliminary to the most fundamental difficulties involved with a policy of selectively nontreating some infants. The fundamental problems center around the criteria used to determine which infants will die and which will live and the mechanism to be used to implement such criteria.

For our purposes the argument for selective nontreatment of some infants can be usefully conceived of as an attempt to state an exception to a general rule or principle involving the saving of lives in a medical context. Usually the basic moral principle of medicine, "do no harm," is construed such that death is the greatest harm. The physician is usually held to account for not saving a life and he or she generally acts on a principle that enjoins one to save a life if that is possible in a given case. We may state a noncontroversial version of such a principle as follows:

> GP: Where it is possible to do so, and especially as it involves one's professional responsibilities, one should choose to save those lives that one can save.

This principle is even stricter in its applications for parents than it is for physicians. A physician going to treat gravely ill individuals at a hospital need not stop and render assistance at the scene of an automobile crash. But if his or her child were involved in the crash, it seems clear that he or she should stop to see that the child does not need him or her more than those in a hospital. It has been cogently argued that parents have a legal duty to provide needed medical care irrespective of the disabilities of the infant; the above example suggests that their moral responsibilities in this regard are somewhat stronger than those of the physicians.

Clearly this general principle has some exceptions that we

regard as acceptable and precise enough to be immune from the criticism I am lodging against selective nontreatment. To save one life while you lose your own may be heroic or saintly but is not generally required of you morally, though many parents believe differently. My formulation is meant to be specifically framed to apply to the medical context where both physician and parent have a somewhat stronger obligation to save the life of the child and where the physician usually can do so and therefore neither physician nor parent is faced with cases involving serious risks to their own lives.

The proponents of selective nontreatment of some newborns would modify this principle with the addition of an exception clause; the GPE would now read:

> GPE: Where it is possible to do so, and especially as it involves one's professional responsibilities one should choose to save those lives that one can save, except when the life saved will be one that is not worth living anyway.

Given the structure of the argument, the crucial issue at stake is obviously to specify criteria for the application of the exception clause such that the exception does not destroy the force of the general principle.[13] Unless proponents of selective nontreatment can provide reasonable, nonarbitrary criteria for the application of the exception clause, it will logically apply to a far broader range of cases in which the general principle of saving a life is thought to apply. In this respect the advocates of GPE may be asking us to accept an exception clause that leads logically to results in particular cases that are seriously at odds with the considered moral convictions and practices of a substantial majority of otherwise well informed and morally sensitive individuals.

Furthermore, the search for such criteria is a direct assault on the fundamental constitutive essence of the liberal regime, without any of the intervening problems of individual liberty that are present when conscious adults seek their own death by suicide or euthanasia. The infant cannot choose for himself or herself; the infant can never have made his or her wishes known by word or deed. Therefore, someone must choose for the infant, must decide that he or she does not deserve the most primitive protection a liberal regime can afford its citizens. The problems with such a judgment are many and we shall detail them shortly. Nevertheless, such a review must not obscure the serious break with essence of liberalism that any such policy represents.

The problem with the revised principle—GPE—is that the exception clause expands easily to cover an almost infinite number of persons who someone else believes have a life not worth living. Essentially this expansiveness can be turned in two directions beyond its applicability to a narrow range of cases involving abnormal newborns. One direction concerns the question of age; the other concerns the question of the extent of the defect necessary for the application of the exception clause. These two directions can be delineated by some cases in each category.

Case I

A. An institution for severely and profoundly retarded persons is faced with an outbreak of a potentially fatal but treatable illness such as pneumonia. Should the physician treat the residents aggressively or merely let those who will die do so in as little pain as possible?

B. In an institution for severely retarded persons, a twelve-year-old multiply handicapped boy begins choking on his food. Should the attendant allow him to choke death?

C. A researcher wishes to find human subjects for an important experiment that may prove fatal to some subjects. He approaches the medical director of a facility for severely handicapped persons and asks that he be allowed to use some of these persons. He states that he will offer substantial monetary compensation to the families of these children and that he will not use any individual whose family objects. Should he be allowed to use these people for his experiment?

It seems clearly more in keeping with our considered moral convictions and practices as well as with the principles on which this regime was founded to say that life should be saved and the experiment prohibited in the cases above. Yet this judgment does not follow from an application of the revised principle [GPE]; in fact the contrary seems to follow. Consider that these institutionalized persons may have precisely the same disabilities as those newborns that may be seriously considered for nontreatment.

Furthermore, at birth we are dealing with a very uncertain prognosis of the future life of the infant. For example, consider the two common congenital disorders, Down's syndrome and spina bifida. In trisomy 21, Down's syndrome, the range of IQ will distribute itself in a bell curve with 50 as the median instead of the normal 100. But this means that, in any population of affected persons, there will be a great variation in phenotype. Some will be only mildly retarded. But it is impossible to discriminate such persons at birth from those who will be at the other end of the spectrum solely on the basis of trisomy 21. Myelomeningocele is even more difficult. Here a majority of these affected—even in the worst prognostic category in terms of the location and size of the lesion—will have essentially normal IQs. Some of these persons will have severe physical handicaps, but how they will respond to this condition is so much a matter of individual temperament and family environment that it is useless to say at birth whether or not they will face much suffering.

However, we have the possibility of a much more accurate evaluation of the life of individual institutional residents. We would thus be in a much better position to make the required judgment about the quality of life of the child without error. In short, if we accept the case for nontreatment of defective newborns, there is at least as strong if not a stronger case for accepting a similar policy for hundreds of thousands of severely retarded and handicapped children and adults being cared for in institutions throughout this country.

This result seems to contradict much of the developing public policy about retarded and handicapped persons. Under the prodding of right-to-treatment cases, much increased effort and expense has been generated for severely retarded persons being cared for in institutions. The presuppositions of such policies are that each retarded person should be given the opportunity to achieve whatever level of development his or her abilities will allow. Such a belief is inconsistent with a judgment that an individual has a life not worth living. If a person has such a life it would appear to be a waste of social resources to provide him or her with the increased help envisioned in these right to treatment policies.

There are still two lines of rebuttal that can be made to this argument that the logical extension of GPE to older children and adults leads to unacceptable results. Both involve attempts to distinguish institutionalized retarded persons from infants so that the policy developed for infants need not logically apply to older children with the same defect. First, it may be claimed that, having treated these children at birth and given repeated care afterward, we have now created a social obligation to support them that is does not extend to newborns.

This maneuver, however, will not sustain the weight put on it. Even if we admitted that, *prima facie,* we ought to follow through on a social commitment to render care, it surely seems that if anything could defeat that obligation an admission that the child has a life not worth living surely would. If he does not have such a life, the case for letting such an infant die collapses. On the other hand, if such a life will be so bad that one ought to die rather than endure it, it seems cruel to force one to live it as a ten-year-old when a means of painlessly releasing the person from his or her misery lies close at hand.

Furthermore, it is difficult to see what kind of obligation initially providing care established. The very provision of care surely will not do. If I take care of you once, I need not do so again unless some agreement exists by the terms of which I should do so. The notion that society, merely by offering care initially, has implied a continuous willingness to do so is short-sighted. The offering of care is based on a perception of the moral standing of the recipient. If the infant had such a status

86

then, why should not a similar infant be accorded the same status now? But if it is maintained that we were wrong in initially giving care, as some of those who argue for selective infanticide do claim, then we still have no reason to compound that error by keeping the severely disabled child alive.

A second argument is that caring for the severely retarded child says something about the moral tenor of our society that we would lose if the cold logic of the above argument were strictly followed. Keeping these children alive and well cared for bears witness to our moral fiber and is justified as such. Unfortunately, this argument cannot be maintained with compelling force. If these children are actually suffering to the extent required to prefer that infants with such problems not be kept alive, then I fail to see the rationale of any such moral example. It seems rather to be a pointless exercise in the prolongation of suffering. If, on the other hand, the way society treats its smallest and weakest members says something very profound about the society, the argument applies with equal and perhaps greater force to the newborn, who likely will have fewer voices to speak for him.

In short there seems to be no way to distinguish the severely disabled newborn from older children with the same handicaps. It seems clear, however, that some of our most basic convictions as a people are involved in those public policies mandating not death but better care for severely retarded and handicapped children and adults. Those who favor the adoption of the revised principle GPE ask for a fundamental reversal of these convictions and the policies based on them. This reversal is, I submit, far more morally dubious than most of the proponents of selective nontreatment have recognized; I doubt that many of them would support it.

Who Will Select

The examples in the first group were basically concerned with the need to be consistent across relevantly similar cases. One could take account of the difficulty they posed by simply accepting the serious consequences for public policy that I have noted and then agreeing with the consistent application of a policy on nontreatment in all relevantly similar cases.

Case II

A. An infant is born with a severe physical disability such as Apert's syndrome which nevertheless leaves him or her with a strong likelihood of being within a normal intelligence range. The infant will need a great deal of extra medical care, without which he or she will die. Should the parents be permitted to withhold such care or should they be advised to do so by the physician?

B. An infant is born with Down's syndrome and with accompanying abnormalities such that she will need an operation in forty-eight hours to save her life. The operation is not risky but it is necessary. Furthermore the child will be left with Down's syndrome, which results in typically moderate, sometimes severe retardation. Should the parents be advised to forgo the operation and let the child die or should they even be permitted to do this?

The cases in our second group raise a much more serious theoretical problem. Here we must specify the criteria for determining what constitutes a life not worth living such that only those cases that one desires to consider for nontreatment actually have treatment withheld, resulting in death. The examples in the first group dealt with the need to be consistent, the ones now under review point to the need to be precise and nonarbitrary in stating the criteria to be used and fair in the application of such criteria.

Often writers favoring selective nontreatment cite extreme examples to justify their position. This is unhelpful, however, until we know just how far toward the normal child or infant the policy of selective nontreatment will be allowed to extend. Should newborns with Down's syndrome be included in a nontreatment policy? What about possibly severe physical abnormalities such as neurofibromatosis which frequently leave the child mentally normal? What about borderline retarded children in large, poor families? Finally what about children born to families with a history of serious physical abuse of their offspring? Unless and until such questions as these are successfully answered the proposals for selective nontreatment fail any modest test of an adequate policy proposal.

In the literature one finds two separate approaches to the problem of specifying, adequately, precise criteria for nontreatment. The first approach attempts to set forth a procedural mechanism by which the decision for nontreatment can be best made. As such it evades the question of when a nontreatment decision should be made by offering instead a rationale for who should make it. In making this maneuver it fails on two counts. First, the specification of adequate criteria is a question that cannot be avoided as we shall shortly see. Second, some of the procedural mechanisms actually proposed are in fact inadequate and some are an open invitation to the worst forms of unfairness. Each of these difficulties can be illuminated if we examine closely a procedural answer that has been advanced in recent years by several authors: reliance on the informed judgment of the parents.[14]

Whether or not parents are capable of making such a judgment as this is a matter of controversy among physicians in the field. Some believe that they are emotionally incapable usually of the requisite judgment, at least in the early period just after learning that they have a defective infant.[15] Unfortunately it is in this early period when some decisions must be made. Nevertheless, some physicians feel that parents must make this decision because they—and no one else—will have to live with it, and also because they are in the best position to know in detail the needs of their family and the abilities of they and the other family members to care for a handicapped child.[16] Despite these claims, the procedure is fraught with difficulties.

To begin with, reliance on this procedure is hardly fair to the infants involved in a range of such cases. If we believe that for some infants death is preferable to life then allowing a supposedly irrational parent to order every possible treatment for a child while allowing another parent to withhold routine therapy from a severely handicapped infant is hardly even minimally fair to the first infant. This is not a farfetched example. For example, it is well known that parental religiosity of the family background of the mother correlates highly with the willingness of the parents to care for a defective child.[17] Those who endorse parental decision making in life or death situations for defective newborns are therefore endorsing a procedure that may make the continued life of the infant dependent on the background beliefs or sentiments of the parents. This result is in bold contradiction to the unanimous result of a long series of court cases and is, I submit, strongly counterintuitive as well.[18]

The fairness of absolute reliance on parental choice is impossible to sustain precisely because parents differ so markedly in what they believe constitutes life not worth living. Moreover the intuitive cogency of the position is also difficult to accept. Even if we agree that parents ought to decide whether they wish a handicapped child to live or die we still need to know the range of cases in which parents will be permitted to make such a decision. As the cases involving religious or quasi-religious groups suggest, there are parents willing to refuse treatment for their children for some questionable reasons. The same may be said of any decision procedure—there are those who will use it for any number of good or bad reasons. Unless we are willing to adopt the unreasonable proposition that parents should have this choice for death respected in every case— for example, when normal children need blood transfusions— then we still need to find an acceptable answer to the question of just when life does become not worth living.

Any scheme which permits discretionary judgment in any context requires for its cogency some clear notion of precisely when the decision maker is to be permitted to exercise his or her discretion and when not. Sometimes we might permit the exercise of discretion in all instances. But this cannot be the case here; otherwise, we would evaporate the category of medical neglect of children. The question cannot be avoided simply by relying on the decision of parents, physicians, hospital committees and courts. The argument made about parental choice applies similarly to all proposed third parties who might render a decision that a given infant ought to die rather than live with one's handicaps.

Nevertheless, the policy of unconstrained parental choice has recently been advanced in two interesting but quite different ways. If successful, either one or both of these arguments might provide the serious defense of parental choice that has been lacking in the literature advocating such a policy. The first argument rests on the observation that whatever the definition of a meaningful life for the child, achieving it will depend on a commitment by the parents to offer adequate care for the child. Hence, it is argued, parents must be allowed to make the decision concerning the use of life saving therapy. Unless the parents believe that the child's life will be meaningful they are unlikely to provide the kind of care that can make it meaningful in any degree. Therefore, their assessment of what constitutes a life worth living ought to be controlling.[19]

This is an interesting move. If successful it would provide a better rationale than anyone else has provided for reliance on parental choice and the supposed unfairness that results therefrom. Unfortunately, however, I believe that the cogency of this position cannot be sustained. The central problem is that the crucial question of a life not worth living cannot be avoided as this argument seeks to do. This can be seen most clearly by considering the fact that the above argument need not apply to a handicapped child at all. If an otherwise normal infant is born to a family with a history of serious mental and physical abuse of their children, ought we to refuse to give medical care simply because the family asserts their inability to offer care and nurture? The suggestion that we ought to allow such a child to die merely because the parents have no commitment to offering quality care is one which I find plainly counterintuitive and a serious departure from the organizing assumptions of our regime. Yet a strict application of this argument seems to lead to this conclusion.

It may be replied that the above argument is only meant to

apply to those cases where a family must decide whether a child with a certain range of handicaps will excessively burden their capacity to offer adequate care. Assert this, however, and my point is granted. For then we would need to know just what the range of such cases is, how far toward the normal child or infant liberty for parental choice will be allowed to extend. If this argument does not entail the proposition that any child can be medically abandoned simply because of parental choice, then we will need to know where the line of demarcation is between these sets of cases. With no reasonable boundaries for parental discretion to choose death over life for their infant, this argument fails.

The policy of unencumbered parental choice has also been advanced along another intriguing line of inquiry in recent years. Again, the focus is on the burden which the care will place on the parents and family. Here, however, the relationship between the presence of burden and the right of parental choice is said to be based on the straightforward claim that we do not typically obligate individuals to bear burdens which are, for them, grave or unbearable or which would preclude their being able to fulfill other serious moral obligations.[20] Furthermore, given the difficulties and biases that will inevitably attend any attempt to judge such burdens as outsiders, we generally permit the individual to judge for oneself when the threshold of what one can bear has been reached. By analogy, it is argued, we ought to permit parents to make the judgment about their ability to care for a handicapped child and hence, determine the care extended to it by the medical staff.

This too is an interesting argument, building from superficially plausible analogies in our common moral life. Unfortunately it breaks down in several places. To begin with, any strict maneuver from moral analogies to public practices will not work. At law individuals are not permitted to absolve themselves of contractual obligations merely on their own say so. An ordered society could not function if they were. There must be some assurance that individuals will fulfill such obligations, even those that become onerous or burdensome.

Still, it might be alleged that the parents of a defective

92

newborn have not undertaken such an obligation. They did not desire a handicapped child and, absent a prior commitment analogous to a contractual obligation, they ought to be free to forsake the child. Strictly speaking, two caveats must be noted here. First, we would have to exclude the fetus from being a person at this point, or it would follow that the parents had made a commitment to care for another human being—a fetus—that they now seek to abandon on their own claim of burdensomeness. Secondly, the parents should not have made an initial decision to offer care else, again, they will be seeking to absolve themselves of a promissory obligation merely on their own say-so.

Even were the initial steps correctly made, two things are wrong with the argument that results. First, parents do not typically have such a right to withhold life-sustaining medical care from a normal child. Therefore, unless we are willing to rewrite a substantial portion of family law and policy we will still need to know the threshold of infant handicap that will permit parents to fail to fulfill their normal obligations without fear of legal reprisal. This of course takes us back where we started with the same judgment about human life which reliance on parental choice was supposed to avoid.

Even in its own restricted moral terms, however, it seems to me that this argument is difficult to sustain. The problem is that my unwillingness to bear a burden allows me no right to destroy the source of the burden. For example, suppose I am asked to carry a box which proves too heavy for me. I am not thereby free to destroy the contents of the box. Similarly I would be remiss in leaving the box in the middle of the street where it would be destroyed by oncoming cars if I could possibly prevent doing so. Nor would I have the right to ask another person not to carry the box, hoping that it will thereby be destroyed by vandals. Consider another case. Suppose I see a man drowning in a river. If the rescue of the man is too great a task for my swimming abilities, I need not undertake it. But I have no right to deny a trained lifeguard the chance to save the man. Having saved the man, however, the lifeguard is not at liberty to turn him over to me for continued care and keeping.

Not having agreed to any such obligation, I have none to fulfill and would not be remiss in refusing to do so.

It seems to me that the situation is not changed when applied to the newborn. I as a parent have no right to secure the death of the infant even if I am correct in my judgment that caring for it is a greater burden than I and my family can bear. The mere fact—if it is a fact—that I cannot care for the child does not mean that the child should not be cared for. At most, one could conclude that I should not be burdened with trying to provide such care. If I have reasonably decided that I am unable to care for the child then public and medical policy should not ask me to care for it, provided that some assessment has been made of the correctness of my judgment regarding the capacity of me and my family to offer adequate care.[21]

At this point the question reverts to one involving the disability of the infant. Since offering care would not now entail burdening one person or family in a degree they cannot withstand, the only reason left for preferring the death of the child would be the quality of the future life of the child. Such a judgment is dealt with in the rest of this chapter. Suffice it to say that we have seen all attempts to rely on parental choice still requiring such a judgment about the life of the child. Unless a policy embodying such a choice, made by one human being for another, will stand up under analysis, reliance on parental discretion in any form cannot be sustained.

Since it is impossible to evade the substantive question about a life not worth living, criteria for determining the quality of life of the newborn to be sufficiently minimal to meet this test must be produced. Several authors have attempted to provide some defining criteria for distinguishing those infants that should be saved from those that should not; for the most part the attempts have been a dismal failure. Some writers content themselves with vague generalities such as the claim that some lives represent a hardship and as such should not be maintained.[22] This of course tells us nothing of what we need to know, since hardship could apply to any life at all. As such it offers no distinguishing principles whatsoever.

Other writers offer almost equally vague descriptions of

94

the life not worth living which some infants are supposedly to be spared. Consider for example Marvin Kohl's argument in which he claims that: "A span of life becomes devoid of meaning roughly when, or to the extend to which, an individual cannot possess goals or when, if he can and does have goals, he believes that they are trivial or impossible to achieve."²³ As a matter of policy, this definition of the *meaningless life,* and Kohl's further proposals for physician actions, are unacceptable. If he means to claim that any goal, no matter how small, is adequate to give life meaning, there will be virtually no infants in the meaningless-life category. Even the most severely defective children can pursue certain aims, especially under the guidance of wise therapists or parents.²⁴

But if he means either

a. that one must consciously possess goals one knows one has or
b. that the goals must not be as minimal as implied above,

then he has offered us a very disturbing and morally offensive description of the lives of hundreds of thousands of profoundly and severely retarded persons. This is especially true if we accept Kohl's position that the active termination of meaningless lives is morally proper.²⁵ Pushed to the further question, "Are we obligated to terminate these lives?" Kohl hedges; undoubtedly, he is aware that he is on the verge of endorsing a program of genocide. The hedge is ineffective. He claims that while one may abhor something, such as ugliness, one is not thereby morally permitted to destroy all that one considers ugly. Why not? Presumably either because they have some other valuable qualities or because someone else subjectively values them. The latter alternative would rule out all infanticide and Kohl cannot be supposed to have intended this result. We are left therefore, with the former alternative.

Unfortunately, this is not much help either. To exclude genocide we would need to know what these overriding qualities are and why some infants have them and some do not. These are questions which Kohl refuses to answer except in the vague terms noted above. In fact I think it would be very difficult for him to do so. He has already maintained that these individuals have meaningless lives and that ending such lives is a morally right act, at least *prima facie*. If a person really does have such a life, would it not be a paradigm of cruelty to inflict continued existence on him or her? If one's life is so worthless that killing him or her would be a positive good, it is difficult to see what considerations could be advanced to keep him or her alive. Hence it is difficult to avoid the conclusion that, except in a very few cases—which Kohl leaves unspecified—all of these lives ought to be ended. Implicitly Kohl has offered a case for the mass elimination of tens of thousands of infants and he has not succeeded in separating himself from the logic of his argument.

Once we move beyond vague generalities, such as those found in Kohl or others of a similar bent, we find three sorts of criteria being proposed in the literature for determining when nontreatment of a newborn is in the best interest of the infant.

1. At the most primitive level it cannot be in a person's best interest to pursue futile courses of action. We may surely presume that medical interventions that will not be successful cannot possibly be in the interest of anyone and may therefore be forsaken. Though obvious in the abstract, this primitive understanding of *best interest* is not nearly so unambiguous in its application as some writers suppose.[26] For example, what counts as futile therapy? Is it one that is only successful in saving the life of the infant in 5 per cent or 10 per cent of the cases? If a treatment is only successful in saving the life of infants in a very few of the cases, then we need to strike a balance between futile therapy and saving life, a balance that is not given but which requires choice in the face of ambiguity. Furthermore, what about therapies that are effective in sustaining life but which cannot be employed indefinitely, such as total parenteral nutrition for short bowel syndrome. Is this futile therapy or not? We often do not know in any certain way the outcome of aggressive therapy beforehand. At some point ambiguity slides into futility; but where it does so is neither obvi-

ous nor unproblematic. The legislation now adopted by Congress, which refers to a class of "virtually futile treatments" that can be withheld, seemingly reflects this uncertainty in its language. Such language implies the very range of uncertainty that we have just noted.

A more serious difficulty arises in cases where the infant has a condition that will eventually prove fatal but not immediately so and a life threatening condition that requires therapy now. For example, infants with trisomy 18 typically have a spectrum of serious abnormalities that will eventually prove fatal: only 10 per cent of such infants survive the first year; 50 per cent die in the first two months. The gravity of their situation seems obvious. But while we may say that they are terminally ill, it is not true that every proposed treatment will be ineffective in alleviating a potential cause of death in a specific instance. We may successfully treat respiratory distress or provide nutrition in the face of gastro-intestinal deformities even though the prognosis remains grim.

What is at stake here is the notion of terminal illness; it seems to me that imminent death clearly is not part of our usual understanding of the term.[27] Patients with degenerative diseases like Alzheimer's disease or Lou Gehrig's disease are surely terminally ill and we commonly refer to them in these terms. Yet death can be two or three years away from the point at which the disease is first diagnosed in the patient. The crucial question seems to me to be whether there is a necessary and sufficient causal relationship between a specific disease state and a fatal outcome. This seems to be what we mean by terminal illness: a specific pathological disorder that necessarily ends in death. In cases where a fatal outcome is not certain we are likely to say that one has a potentially or possibly fatal illness. In cases of genetic disease where the phenotypical expression is delayed, such as Huntington's chorea, we do not say that the pathological process has started until the phenotype begins to present itself.

2. At least the futility standard is clear in the abstract and

universally acknowledged on all sides. But it does not really reach the most interesting cases such as those noted above. Here much dispute has ensued. Next to futility the most widely heard claim is that best interest for the infant can be explicated in terms of pain and suffering. If the life of the infant will be filled with pain and suffering, his or her interest supposedly will be best served if he or she is allowed to die. The new legislation does not go as far as this, for it merely permits the withholding of virtually futile treatments that would be inhumane for the infant. Clearly however, many physicians and parents want to adopt a broader pain and suffering standard and would be prone to do so under this language.

The problem with any such standard is that it combines two very different sorts of things: pain and suffering. Though often related, neither one is necessary or sufficient to produce the other. Pain is a physiological response to a perceived injury, a response either at the subconscious, thalamic level or at the conscious level of the cerebral cortex where it is open to introspection and interpersonal disclosure; this is when I can say to myself or others that "I am in pain."[28] To be capable of experiencing pain, therefore, one need not be conscious, a fact that is acknowledged in the accepted criteria for distinguishing comatose persons from those who are brain dead. The response of the person to known painful stimuli is a crucial criterion for distinguishing these cases in clinical practice.[29]

Suffering, on the other hand, is an emotional response, a felt anguish in the face of our inability to sustain our present happiness or reach our desired goals. In other words, suffering entails a sense of loss. In a fine recent essay Eric Cassel has written: "Most generally suffering can be defined as the state of severe distress associated with events that threaten the intactness of the person."[30] The person's concept of himself or herself, of who one is and what one can do if one chooses is threatened and with the threat one suffers.

98

From this widely acknowledged understanding of suffering, two necessary conditions for suffering are apparent: sentience and the perception of loss. Sentience is not necessary for one to be in pain but it is necessary for one to suffer. Moreover, unless one can sense a loss or incompleteness in one's person or capacities, one cannot suffer. It seems uncontroversial to say that this perception of loss occurs when one knows the difference between what one is and what one would like to be. A quadraplegic like Ellen Bouvia suffers because she knows how life could be if she were normal. Her sense of the absence of a cherished capacity is the source of suffering. If one cannot sense that difference, one cannot, I think, really be said to suffer.

Once distinguished, two points about suffering seem obvious. First, the suffering of others is notoriously opaque to us: we very often simply do not know whether another person is suffering and especially not the extent or severity of his or her suffering. For example, we may reasonably presume that a person is in pain if he or she has a condition that typically produces pain in normal human beings, such as an open wound. But we cannot so presume suffering. Without self-disclosure, it is extremely difficult to know how much anyone suffers. What will cause suffering to one person will not to another, and each person's suffering threshold is likely to be an extremely personal compound of familial influence, personal history, religious faith, and anticipation of the future. These are the very things that we know least about in our encounters with others.

Second, it seems eminently reasonable and supported by empirical data that those persons who suffer most with handicaps are those who are most nearly normal in intelligence. Severe physical handicaps by themselves are more likely to produce suffering in a person of normal intelligence than in a person who is severely retarded. At the very least, we have no reason to presume suffering when people can neither disclose their suffering nor be expected to experience the absence of something they desire. It seems quite implausible to believe that someone who does

not know about the capacities of normal adults, as profoundly retarded persons may not, will suffer from their
lack.[31]

If the distinction between pain and suffering is made
in this manner, it seems clear that pain is relevant to a best-
interest test for abnormal newborns but that suffering cannot be. We can presume that the infant has an interest in
being free from pain and that, where no larger therapeutic
purpose is served, uncontrolled pain is not in his or her
interest. We would not, I think, find it unreasonable for
adults to refuse continued life-sustaining therapy in such
cases and we cannot treat infants differently.

Suffering is an entirely different matter. Since suffering requires a consciousness of loss or difference, we are
faced with the anomalous situation that the possibility of
suffering is likely to increase as the person approaches the
range of normal intelligence. But these are precisely the
cases in which no one seems to prefer death over life. Even
such a radical advocate of selective nontreatment as Joseph
Fletcher wants to limit euthanasia to those infants at the
lowest end of the IQ spectrum.[32] Furthermore, as intelligence increases so does the capacity to give meaning to
one's disabilities or to alter one's desires, either of which
reduce or alter suffering. This can occur in many ways such
as counselling or religious commitment but whatever the
manner in which meaning is engendered, it clearly seems
wildly implausible to prefer nontreatment and death to the
pursuit of meaning and the reduction of suffering when
the infant is older.

3. The most controversial criterion that is sometimes
brought up in a best-interest test for newborn intensive
care is that having to do with the possession of some "higher" human characteristics by the infant.[33] Though notoriously difficult to specify and open to much dispute, such
characteristics are often asserted to be essential in the consideration of such cases of abnormal newborns. Of the
available formulations of such criteria, those that are most
frequently noted have to do with the capacity or potential

capacity of the infant to enter human relationships with others. In his now classic article, Richard McCormick defined such a position in the following terms:

> life is not a value to be preserved in and for itself. To maintain that would commit us to a form of medical vitalism that makes no human or Judeo-Christian sense. It is a value to be preserved precisely as a condition for other values. . . . Since these other values cluster around and are rooted in human relationships, it seems to follow that life is a value to be preserved only insofar as it contains some potentiality for human relationships. When in human judgment this potentiality is totally absent or would be, because of the condition of the individual, totally subordinated to the mere effort for survival, that life can be said to have achieved its potential. If these reflections are valid, they point in the direction of a guideline that may help in decisions about sustaining the lives of grossly deformed and deprived infants. That guideline is the potential for human relationship associated with the infant's condition.[34]

In a fine recent essay, philosopher John Arras offered another version of this same notion:

> The presence or absence of such characteristics as the ability to think, to communicate, to give and receive love, seems to be highly relevant from a moral point of view. . . . The ethical principle that justifies this standard is the proposition that biological human life is only a relative good. In the absence of certain distinctly human capacities—for self-consciousness and relating to other people—the usual connection between biological life and our notion of the good is effectively severed . . . the absence of fundamental human capacities can render a life valueless, both to its possessor and to others.[35]

However widely held such relational criteria seem to be, fatal ambiguities lurk here. These are not ambiguities in the application of such a standard to particular cases, but rather in the relational standard itself. Two versions seem to present themselves: a sentience version and a self-consciousness version. The sentience version would hold that the necessary and sufficient relationship to meet the standard is constituted if:

1. both parties are human beings, and
2. they enter into a discriminate relationship in which A appears to know that he is in the presence of B.

The self-consciousness version clearly requires more. Just what this "more" may be is difficult to specify. For example, Arras writes of the "ability to think, communicate, to give and receive love"; McCormick writes of "human relationships" in a manner that seemed to imply something more than the very minimal standards of the sentience version. What seems to be at stake in all of these formulations is the consciousness of the individual as an individual with goals and plans in relation to others. In other words it is not enough for A to know that he or she is in the presence of B. One must know that he or she and B are human beings who relate to each other as independent selves with cognitive capacities of the distinctively human, symbol manipulating sort.

Once these two versions of the relational standard are identified, it seems clear that only the sentience version can possibly form the basis of public policy for newborn intensive care. The alternative broader formulations are so loosely framed as to be incapable of defining an actual range of exceptions to the rule mandating care that do not evacuate the force of the rule itself. Either far too many exceptions are justified or none at all beyond the comatose infant.

Consider for example, the formulation of this standard offered by Albert Jonson and Michael Garland in a well-known essay.

> Intensive care may, in the context of certain life conditions, appear harmful. These conditions are identified as inability to survive infancy, inability to live without severe pain and inability to participate at least minimally in human experience.[36]

The first two conditions, inability to live even with treatment and inability to live without severe pain have been addressed above.[37] It is with the third case that problems arise.

102

The authors realize this but in attempting to explain what they mean they simply add to the confusion.

> The third condition is perhaps, the most controversial and therefore needs some explanation. Judgment that an infant is unable to participate in human experience requires projection on the basis of indirect measurements. One must be able to say that there is no reasonable expectation that the infant will ever be able to respond affectively or cognitively to attention and caring or to engage in communication with others. The criterion has to do with presence or absence of capacity, not merely with degrees of deviation from the normal.[38]

The problem with both of these versions of the criterion is that they simply won't do in practice, as a public or medical policy. If these authors mean that any ability for human relationships or for response to human caring is sufficient, then the stated criteria will exclude almost no infants. Even the most profoundly retarded child has some capacity for responding to human care and attention. This is true even in cases of severe physical handicap and where the capacity for coherent speech is nonexistent. Such a result, in which no infants are selected for nontreatment, cannot be presumed to be the policy intended by these authors since they both give examples of nontreatment that go far beyond such a guideline.

On the other hand, if they wish to go further then they include in the criteria hundreds of thousands of severely or profoundly retarded individuals. Consider for example Jonson and Garland's phrase, "respond affectively and cognitively to human attention." If they really mean that the individual must have capacities for both affective and cognitive response then very few profoundly retarded persons currently being cared for in institutions will have the requisite cognitive ability. It would appear therefore that they are willing to sanction the nontreatment of all of these individuals. If a life threatening condition confronts these profoundly retarded persons, the morally proper thing to do would be to let them die quickly.

Of course medical care in the strict sense may not be all that many of these children need to save their lives. For example many of the multiply handicapped children have trouble in feeding themselves. It is not an uncommon occurrence to have such children choke on their food. There is little difference between such a life threatening situation and those involving the respirator or other forms of medical therapy. Followed consistently, therefore, the advice offered by Jonson and Garland and McCormick would be to stand by and let the child choke to death. It seems to me that any policy that results in such a morally repugnant conclusion is fundamentally wrong and must be abandoned, especially a public standard of judgment.

If we give up the hopeless quest for these sorts of criteria based on notions of "relational capacity" or "cognitive self-consciousness," will a standard based on sentience be adequate or acceptable. Such a standard, based simply on sentience, has fewer obvious problems of vagueness, expansiveness or fairness than the alternatives. Moreover it does seem to reflect a very widely held consensus about how we ought to treat permanently comatose individuals, that is, they need not be kept alive by artificial means.

Space does not permit a lengthy analysis of such a standard but we can note three arguments for it that might not entail the conclusions about a life not worth living which now concern us. First, as a practical matter, infants who are permanently comatose almost surely have conditions that are either certain to or likely to lead to their death.[39] Secondly, one might argue that sentience is a necessary condition of being a human being; as such, the comatose person would have no human moral standing. This however is at odds with our common way of referring to comatose individuals and might lead to the permission of inhumane or cruel treatment of those who can still feel pain. This is clear because one of the cases reported by Duff and Campbell in their important 1973 paper involved the classic situation of Down's syndrome and intestinal atresia. They permitted the parents to refuse the surgery necessary for feeding the child.

Thirdly, one might argue that the possession of or capacity to exercise rights is dependent on the capacity to experience the consequences of exercising the rights in question. In other

104

words, the capacity to take an interest in something might be crucial to being able to have a right regarding that thing. Since the comatose person cannot know of life at all, especially a comatose infant who has never known it, he cannot properly be said to have an interest or a right in this regard at all. As such, no moral wrong is done in not saving his life. On this view, the possession of rights exists along a spectrum; while the comatose person may experience pain or even hunger, and may have rights based on such capacities, he may not have other capacities necessary to having other rights.[40]

In my view there is much to be said in practice for a sentience standard, even if a completely convincing rationale is lacking. This is especially true given the very dismal prognosis of almost all comatose infants and adults. At the very least it seems to reflect a widespread sentiment that can be specified in relatively precise and inelastic terms and which need not lead to characterizations of the comatose individual that might justify or permit inhumane or painful forms of "care."

Criteria: Means of Treatment

In light of the difficulties we have seen with attempts to develop a disease oriented set of quality-of-life criteria for determining when an infant is afflicted with a "life not worth living," some writers have adopted the treatment oriented ordinary/extraordinary means terminology for delineating just which infants ought to be allowed to die. On this view treatment is optional if it is "extraordinary" or "heroic" and mandatory if it is "ordinary." In my view this argument fails because, in practice, it ends up being indistinguishable from the "quality of life" argument to which it is supposedly superior.

This can be seen if we consider the conclusions of one important advocate of this argument. In his book, Leonard Weber proposes that every handicapped infant should be treated *unless*

1. the treatment is not likely to be successful.

or

105

2. the treatment imposes an excessive burden on the child—for example, he or she can expect a very long period of intensive fighting for life or the treatment itself results in a severe and permanent handicap.

or

3. the treatment imposes an excessive burden on the family.[41]

There are several reasons why this approach must be rejected for policy purposes. First, the key concept, "excessive burden," is nowhere defined precisely, either by Weber or in the Roman Catholic literature from which this concept is taken.[42] One pores over that literature in vain seeking clearly expressed, coherent definitions of such a concept that could be useful in forming public policies on the question at hand. Set in a different context, this literature is almost a dull replay of the life not worth living discussion which we have already reviewed.

The reason that it reads like a replay is that, in fact, it is largely the same argument. The extraordinary-means position does not avoid the problems of the life-not-worth-living judgment because it too is forced to render the same judgment and is therefore faced with all the insoluble problems that such a move entails.

In this regard, McCormick is absolutely correct when he notes that the terms *ordinary* and *extraordinary means* are nothing more than code words denoting the moral status of various medical acts in a given case; for example, an NG tube would be ordinary in this case, intubation would not. He is also correct in arguing that, as traditionally used, this language is patently a quality-of-life judgment, especially insofar as hardship or burden on the patient is allowed to determine an extraordinary and therefore optional form of treatment. In most cases the actual treatment itself is not difficult or burdensome; what is difficult is the life of the patient during or after treatment. Travel to a different climate—a favorite example of older writers—is today hardly onerous or burdensome itself. What made it optional for

106

these writers was its expense and its uprooting of the person from familial and social surroundings.[43]

Consider in this regard just Weber's fairly standard presentation of the position. He claims that a treatment may be withheld if it imposes an excessive burden on the child. The example is a treatment which in itself, handicaps the child.[44] But again the unanswered question contains the real payoff—how handicapped must the child become as a result of the treatment before that treatment becomes optional. Is mere nonambulation enough? In his classic paper on treatment for spina bifida Lorber maintained that the children who were worst off were those who were mentally normal or close to normal but who were confined to a nonambulatory state. They knew what they were missing and suffered greatly as a result.[45] Would such a situation be excessive burden and the amputation of diseased legs therefore optional for the parents of a small child? For a small child any attempt to determine how he would react to such circumstances would be largely guesswork. What we would be left with is the parental assessment of what they believe a worthwhile life to be. This of course brings the circle home again and leaves us where we started with the life-not-worth-living judgment in the beginning.

This point becomes even clearer when we examine Weber's third circumstance in which extraordinary treatment is optional. Here he proposes that family burdens are, by themselves, sufficient sometimes to render the proposed treatment optional. Such a claim has been fully discussed above and it seems to me that the conclusion reached there is correct, whether we are discussing the financial or other burdens imposed by the treatment itself or the burden of caring for the child. In fact, it appears that these two considerations are deeply intertwined. Consider again Weber's example of an operation that handicaps a child yet saves his or her life. In such a case is a family at liberty to decide that they will be too gravely burdened by the results of operation to permit it to proceed? Weber would seem to be committed to saying yes at this point.[46] If so, he must be willing either to permit indiscriminate parental choice in these cases or he must produce the criteria necessary for judging the correctness of a parental choice. The only way out is for Weber to produce a clearly expressed, tightly developed statement of just what kind of handicap will pose an excessive burden. But such a judgment about a life not worth living is one that Weber consistently refuses to render.

Weber's reply to these sorts of arguments is to insist that he is referring to those types of situations in which the treatment itself, not the handicap, leaves the child or the family excessively burdened. This distinction is largely spurious. In fact, Weber himself makes this point obvious when he notes that a treatment is burdensome to the child if it leaves him or her severely handicapped. In such a case, the reason for refusing treatment would be the handicap—and hence quality of life—of the child after therapy. Much the same, it seems to me, must be said of a possible excessive burden on a family. If a family regards a nonambulatory, bowel incontinent handicap as more than they can bear, are they permitted to refuse therapy that will leave a child in this condition? Weber's answer, I believe, must be yes. If so, I think it is spurious to claim that something is going on here other than a family judging that a child with a certain handicap will be more than they can bear. The therapy is optional because it leads to handicaps for the child, which are more than this family can withstand. Therapy may therefore be withheld and the child let die.

In short, the extraordinary means maneuver solves none of the important problems encountered in shaping public policy regarding the nontreatment of sick infants and children. It may even add new ones with its longstanding insistence that excessive burden to a family will justify the death of the child and its need to define both an excessively burdensome treatment per se in such variables as cost, length, difficulty, pain, discomfort, and so forth, and its need to define the degree of handicap that will justify a decision not to treat.

The Role of the Federal Government

The case for selective infanticide or nontreatment fails as an acceptable policy. None of the arguments on its behalf are plausible nor do the proffered policy formulations show any promise of avoiding serious contradictions and difficulties. The questions that remain are those regarding the proper formulation of and locus of authority for setting forth a policy of saving the lives of infants irrespective of their supposed quality.

This issue has been brought to a head in recent years when the Federal Government sought to adopt regulations designed to prevent discrimination against handicapped infants in neonatal intensive care. The federal involvement came in the wake of a widely publicized case in which a Bloomington, Indiana infant with Down's syndrome and intestinal atresia was deprived of surgery to correct the atresia. As a result the infant could not be fed and died.[47] This case was so patently unacceptable and so clearly a failure of state courts and law enforcement that the Department of Health and Human Services felt compelled to act. It acted under authority of section 504 of the Rehabilitation act of 1973 that forbids Federal financial assistance to any institution that discriminates against the handicapped.[48] In this case the government interpreted its mandate broadly—though correctly—and put hospitals on notice that such discrimination was unlawful and could result in a termination of federal money going to the hospital.[49] Since few hospitals could survive without federal grants, payments for medicare or medicaid or other forms of Federal assistance, this was a particularly effective enforcement measure insofar as hospitals were concerned.[50]

The key to the government's position rested on how it chose to define the discrimination it sought to punish. For these purposes the government chose to define unlawful discrimination as occurring if:

1. the withholding is based on the fact that the infant is handicapped; and
2. the handicap does not render the treatment or nutritional sustenance medically contraindicated.[51]

At this point two questions obviously present themselves: is this an adequate rule? and should the federal government set it forth and enforce it? First, it must be admitted that this rule leaves much to be desired. The second clause—the exception—is, as one sympathetic critic has noted, "so vague that it is unintelligible."[52] The phrase *medically contraindicated* could mean contraindicated because the child is so handicapped that he is unlikely to have a life worth living after treatment or because one's handicap renders it unlikely that one's life can be saved even with aggressive therapy. From the text itself one really does not know what interpretation is intended. But this uncertainty is fatal to the rule as it stands since it offers no clinically useful guidance to those faced with decisions regarding the care of individual handicapped infants.

If one really means to exclude quality of life considerations usually unnecessary in the decisions in these sorts of cases one should say so plainly: "no child shall be deprived of life-saving medical care, irrespective of the nature and extent of his or her handicap or the supposed quality of his or her prospective life." Such a statement would be tighter and, I believe, clearer than that initially proposed by HHS. At the time, however, it was not clear that HHS had authority to issue such a broad regulation regarding the role of quality of life considerations in medical decision making under the authority of a law designed to prevent discrimination against the handicapped. It was already stretching its mandate to take the action it took. Soon the federal courts struck down that regulation. The precise ground on which the courts struck down the regulation was that the secretary of HHS had attempted to issue the interim final regulation under provisions of federal law that provided for very brief periods of notice and comment by parties affected by these regulations. The court found that no justification existed for invoking these emergency provisions. However, in dicta the court added comments that tended to agree with the plaintiffs on the private nature of these decisions.[53]

The other legal and policy response to the Bloomington tragedy were laws enacted by several states that were specifically designed to prevent such deprivations of life saving medical care. Generally, these laws held that:

1. no child should be deprived of life saving medical care irrespective of quality of life judgments,

110

2. when a family refuses consent for such care the physician or the hospital must report the child as neglected and.
3. a licensed physician may provide life saving care in such a case without liability when a delay in legal resolution of the case would endanger the child's life.[54]

A detailed analysis of these statutes is beyond the scope of this chapter but two observations are in order. First, these statutes are generally clearer and more precise in their crucial sections than were the federal regulations. For example, the Louisiana statute reads:

> No minor child, from the moment of live birth, shall be intentionally deprived of any medical or surgical care by his or her parent, physician or any other person when such medical or surgical care is necessary to attempt to save the life of the child, in the opinion of a physician exercising competent medical judgment despite the opinion of the child's parent or parents, the physician or others that the quality of the child's life would be deficient should the child live.[55]

In this respect, the state laws give more guidance to practitioners with fewer loopholes and are therefore better as policy than the federal regulations. Unfortunately, however, these substantial virtues of the state legislation are almost all lost in the various exception clauses that some of them contain, clauses that evacuate the clear force of the rule itself. For example, in one statute the exclusion of quality of life factors in the crucial operative clause is clear and precise. But this clarity is immediately obscured by the exclusion of permanently comatose infants from the sanctions against the use of quality of life standards in decision making for these infants.[56] Such an exception is not made to rest on a prognosis of likely survival but appears to be derived from quality of life factors that were supposedly excluded in the previous section. Again, the relevant point is that if one wishes to prevent discrimination against some infants because of their supposedly low quality of life, then one ought to do it in clear language.

111

These various legislative and policy responses to tragedies such as that in Bloomington engendered substantial critical commentary. Some of it was focused soundly on the lack of clarity in the crucial operative sections of the federal regulations or the contradictions such as have just been noted in the state legislative remedies that were hastily enacted after the Bloomington case.[57] Other criticisms, especially from the American Medical Association, amounted to the proposition that these should remain private decisions made by physicians and family members alone. The physicians were particularly bothered by the hot line feature of the federal regulations—it required that a notice of the regulation be posted in newborn intensive care units with an accompanying number where suspected violations could be reported to the government, which would then undertake an emergency investigation of the case and intervene as necessary. The physicians especially asserted that this constituted a federal invasion in a very delicate and private matter and was only designed to have an *in terrorem* effect on physician behavior, that is it was designed to terrorize physicians into providing aggressive medical care irrespective of other considerations.[58]

In some important respects these claims are wrong. The proposition that these are private decisions between a physician and a family simply will not stand up. Parents do not own their children or hold plenary power over their lives and in the common law they have never been vested with the private authority to determine whether their children live or die, a judgment found in a hundred years of the development of child-neglect laws. To say that parents and physicians may conspire freely to bring about the death of children who are simply unwanted because of their handicaps represents such a departure from our legal, political, and moral tradition that it simply cannot be the basis of acceptable policy.

The claims about the *in terrorem* effect of the law and its hot line feature fare no better. All law, especially criminal law, engenders action in accord with its provisions precisely because fear of punishment deters substantial deviations from acceptable behavior. If the hot line is sound as policy and necessary as an enforcement measure, the fact that it uses fear of punishment to deter discrimination is surely not a reason to reject it.

In response to these various criticisms, the Department of Health and Human Services began negotiations with groups representing the rights of the disabled, the right-to-life organizations and the American Academy of Pediatrics. This resulted in a revised set of regulations, approved by these groups, issued in January of 1984. After this too was struck down by the courts as being beyond the power of the Federal Government under current law, the revised regulations became the basis of new legislation passed in the summer of 1984 and endorsed by most of the leading organizations in the field except the American Medical Association.[59]

The revised legislation differs fundamentally from the versions that preceded it. Essentially it is an amendment to earlier legislation in which Congress provided funding for state child abuse and neglect agencies if the states would adopt federally mandated standards for defining and intervening in abuse and neglect cases. The amendments set forth a standard for defining medical neglect in neonatal medicine and leave enforcement in the hands of state agencies who have an established authority to intervene in neglect cases. Gone is any federal involvement, including the hot line.

This general framework is much preferable to earlier versions. The earlier versions set forth the terms of direct federal involvement, but in fact the government enforcement mechanisms were at best limited and morally dubious. Even granting the government the power it sought, its capacity to punish offenders and deter offenses was limited to cutting off funding to hospitals where discriminatory practices occurred. This punishes the hospital, and indirectly other patients and third-party payors, for wrongs committed by physicians and parents. Neither the hospital nor the federal government can compel a physician to operate or a parent to consent to an operation. We would not have it otherwise. Hospitals should not be empowered to force physicians to operate without independent review of the merits of the case, nor should we empower the federal government to seek court authorization for an operation, clearly making an exception to the substantial body of abuse and neglect cases already handled by state law and agencies.

Secondly, the new legislation provides a substantive standard defining neglect in these cases. The essential proposition is a presumption in favor of saving or sustaining the life of the infant; furthermore, the actual or anticipated handicaps of the infant are unacceptable bases for nontreatment decisions. The exceptions to this general rule are threefold. Treatment may be withdrawn or withheld:

1. if the treatment is futile, that is, cannot save the life of the child,
2. is virtually futile and inhumane, that is, highly unlikely to save the life of the infant and in itself painful, discomforting, or risky in the circumstances, and
3. if the infant is permanently comatose.[60]

Thirdly, the new legislation encourages, but does not mandate, the formation of hospital bioethics committees that can review cases and make recommendations. Initially the American Academy of Pediatrics proposed that committee review be mandatory in every case where the withdrawal or withholding of care would likely result in the death of the infant. The compromises reached with administrators and clinicians wary of such committees was a strong encouragement but not a legal mandate.

Though only "encouraged" in the actual text of the legislation, the regulation strongly supports the establishment of hospital bioethics committees.[61] This is an important concession. No statute can define in advance the appropriate resolution to every case. There will always need to be judgments made, judgments that are sometimes ambiguous and imprecise.[62] Moreover, state agencies charged with investigating suspected cases of neglect simply cannot be expected to review every case in every hospital. It is even more absurd to believe that an already overburdened court system could conduct such a wide ranging review as may be necessary in these cases. What is needed, therefore, is a mechanism for reviewing all cases where nontreatment is contemplated, not just some few cases that

114

happen to come to the attention of state agencies. Moreover, even when the state agencies become involved they will still need to rely on the very expertise that can be part of the committee process from the beginning. Surely the committees will need to be backed up with the actions of state agencies and orders from courts where particular cases require it. But the consensus is correct, committee review of every case is the best mechanism for advancing the very interests that must be at the center of the decision-making process: those of the infant.

Finally, I think that the one truly meritorious feature of the original regulations was the one most criticized by physicians: the hot line. Physicians and families are undertaking awesome decisions about the lives of the weakest human beings among us, decisions about which law cannot be silent or indifferent. Those who decide ought to remember the seriousness of what they do and the potential injustices that may be involved, injustices that law must deter. Moreover, a simple notice regarding state neglect law with a number to call to report violations would seem to be appropriate and even mandatory as an enforcement tool. The institutions within which these decisions are made and carried out are places of privacy and confidentiality, features that breed the silent injustices that now occur. A notice of legal standards and remedies and a listing of where suspected violations may be reported is not more onerous than similar notices regarding discrimination on the job and, given the seriousness of the potential harms involved, even more mandatory.

Conclusion

It has been said that one measure of a community's concern for its members is found in the way it treats those who are abnormal through no fault of their own. Seen from this angle, the writers we have discussed in this chapter would have us endorse a policy that prefers death to life for some of our smallest citizens, even where extra care could make a difference in the quality of their lives. Infants cannot speak for themselves; they cannot assert their rights against the intrusions of others.

They are totally at the mercy of other human beings to protect and care for them. In this chapter we have seen the case made by those who wish to hedge our historic commitment to these infants, to tie it to some supposed qualities that the infant has or does not have. The confusions and contradictions in the various arguments themselves are surely enough to render the case utterly insufficient for the task it has undertaken. Nevertheless, we must not let the ineptness of a given argument detract us from the central fact: these authors wish us to embark on a public policy that represents a fundamental departure from the organizing principles of the regime itself.

It is true that some infants must die. Their afflictions are too much for even the most skilled medical care. Often death may be the best result. It is also true that often we are not at all certain about the results of aggressive medical care, whether it will save the life of the infant or not. But admitting such sad yet necessary facts is far different from the wholesale infanticide programs logically entailed in the arguments reviewed in this chapter. The moral and political consensus that once protected the infant is breaking down, just as it has broken down for the fetus. But the breakdown of this consensus is hardly to be welcomed by anyone seriously concerned with the future of our society. For this breakdown is perhaps the most serious of all departures from our organizing principles as a community. To welcome that break is to welcome the brave new world that awaits us without the commitment to equal worth which has defined our polity from the beginning.

CHAPTER FOUR

Euthanasia

Introduction

The discussion of euthanasia and the right to die has erupted in our society during the last decade. In hundreds of articles in medical journals, from prestigious publications to specialized quarterlies, it has been discussed with vigor. Journalists have popularized the issues in scores of articles and books. Lawyers have drafted statutes dealing with it and have themselves argued both real and hypothetical cases. Philosophers and theologians have edited anthologies and examined the questions involved in numerous forums.[1]

Legislatures and courts have reflected this activity of the popular and professional press. As this is written more than twenty states since 1971 have revised their legal definition of death to include as dead those persons who have permanent death of the whole brain, even though their vital signs are maintained mechanically.[2] Again, many states have legalized various mechanisms whereby an individual acting for himself, or sometimes a family acting for a member, might secure the removal of life-preserving medical care;[3] in the last five years, numerous other state legislatures have considered similar legislation.[4] The slender margins by which some of these measures were defeated indicate that the number of states with such laws is bound to increase. In still other states, the courts have effectively legislated on the question: they have provided ways for families to refuse medical care for an incompetent member.

The flash point of this discussion was the enormous pouring forth of learned and popular opinion regarding the plight of the young woman from New Jersey, Karen Ann Quinlan. The facts of this case are simple. On the night of April 15, 1975, Karen ceased breathing for at least two fifteen minute periods. The exact cause of these episodes was never fully determined but the result was tragic. Karen went into a coma from which she never recovered. On learning that their daughter had no chance for recovery, the Quinlans asked the attending physicians and the hospital to remove the respirator that presumptively kept Karen alive. They did so with the complete assurance from their Roman Catholic religious authorities that they were acting in accord with the teachings of the church in which they devoutly believed. Believing that such an act would result in Karen's death, the physicians refused; the hospital administrator supported their refusal.[5]

Faced with this situation the Quinlans petitioned for guardianship over their adult daughter and for the right as guardians to withdraw medical care in her behalf. The lower court granted their petition for guardianship but denied that there was any constitutional or common law ground for a right to die and thus rejected the central contention and desire of the Quinlans. On appeal the state's highest court held for the Quinlans on all points. But when Karen was removed from the respirator, she did not stop breathing as everyone had expected. She remained alive for nine years, permanently comatose, kept alive by nourishment through a tube and by antibiotics to ward off the infections that would surely kill her otherwise.[6]

The tragic circumstances of Miss Quinlan's life and the

slow pace of its consideration by the courts directed attention to the situation as emblematic of a tragic choice that parents, court, and all the conscious living face. Were her parents right or wrong? Should they also remove the feeding tube or the antibiotics? Were the arguments of the physicians or the hospital sound? Should society now permit the Quinlans to kill their daughter in some quick and painless way, rather than force them to let her die slowly from infection or starvation?

Since Karen had never made her wishes known precisely, the question of her autonomy could not possibly be a coherent part of the consideration of her case. What was at stake was the propriety of her parents' decision of what would be the most humane choice on her behalf. While it may be that the law would have traditionally respected her autonomous choice in medical matters, it was not at all clear that her parents should have had the power over her life and death that they sought.

Such ambiguity remains. As we shall see in this chapter, the attempts by courts and commentators to make allowance in law and public policy for the actions the Quinlans wished to undertake have by and large resulted only in inadequate or plainly incoherent rationales and vague, dangerously elastic proposals for statutory regulation and medical practice.

History of Modern Euthanasia Movement

The sad case of Miss Quinlan and the commentary it evoked did not occur in a vacuum. For centuries there have been sporadic discussions of what care one should offer to the gravely ill and of the obligations of their physicians. In the twentieth century, the question of euthanasia in all its many forms moved from the back pages of little read treatises to the front pages of medical, ethical, religious, and popular journals.[7]

The founding of the British Euthanasia Society in 1932 served as a catalyst for bringing the issues to public attention in Great Britain; the 1936 founding of its American counterpart spread the concern to the United States. The British society brought before the House of Lords a bill authorizing the active mercy killing of anyone who desired it but it failed, as did a similar bill introduced in Nebraska in 1938 at the request of the American committee.[8]

For the next two decades, the issue remained dormant as a matter of law and public policy. The policies of the Nazis were so abhorrent that few would defend practices that appeared at all similar. Nevertheless, the increasing distance from the horrors of Nazi practice as well as the extraordinary advances of medicine in the postwar period combined to reopen the discussion of euthanasia in the late 1950s and 1960s.

Williams's *The Sanctity of Life and the Criminal Law*

The appearance of Glanville Williams's provocative book, *The Sanctity of Life and the Criminal Law,* and rejoinders to it by several important critics broke the silence forcefully in 1959.[9] Williams frankly advocated active mercy killing of any adult who requested it, provided only that two physicians certified that one suffered from an "incurable illness" that will either cause one "severe distress" or render one "incapable of leading a rational existence." More recently, other writers have advocated such a position; their contributions are discussed below.[10]

Williams based his case on three arguments. First, inconsistency in the law as written and as applied led to uncertainty among the very people whose actions ought to be governed by some legal structure.[11] The law, he argued, cannot continue to proscribe mercy killing and then effectively look the other way when it occurs. Secondly, the case against euthanasia legislation is inseparably connected to religious convictions about the sanctity of life and human prerogative to take it.[12] Such a connection renders the current law deeply suspect as the basis of policy in a secular regime.[13] Thirdly, the failure to enact legislation to permit mercy killing forces individuals to lead lives of misery and suffering.[14]

Of these only the last is telling. Williams's claim that the law is inconsistent in application is one that applies to almost all criminal law, especially since most criminals are not caught; for example, few if any professional hit men are ever caught. Does this mean that we should stop regulating such behavior because of inconsistency between the law as written and the law as applied? The argument about religiousness fares no better. Most legislation touches on the religious claims of some group; race relations give a good example. Surely Williams would not want to claim that all attempts to outlaw overt racial segregation were wrong because they involved the state in enforcing one religious view against another that held that segregation was ordained by God.

Kamisar's Analysis of Williams's Proposal

The most extended reply to his position appeared shortly thereafter in a classic and often reprinted article by Yale Kamisar.[15] Kamisar produced substantial nonreligious objections to mercy killing proposals, as Williams himself admitted.[16] This fact renders the religiousness argument unpersuasive. Kamisar made two replies to Williams basic argument. First, he suggested that there was a real possibility of mistakes or abuse under the suggested policy in which either:

1. the required diagnosis is wrong or
2. the patient will be allowed to make a "choice" when he or she is so under the influence of pain-killing drugs that competency to choose is doubtful.[17]

Secondly, Kamisar argued that the machinery created under the proposal would be extended to cover other classes of persons, such as the retarded and the chronically insane, who meet the standard of "irrational existence" but who cannot consent.[18]

Crucial issues are at work here, especially in Kamisar's second argument, a version of the so-called "wedge principle"; but the statement of the issues is not compelling. Kamisar chose to liken the maneuver to legalize mercy killing to measures adopted in early Nazi Germany; he feared that the rest would follow in due course. Thus Kamisar implied that untenable consequences would follow any attempt to enact legislation such as that proposed by Williams.

Critique of Kamisar

But this statement of the argument is easily refuted by pointing out that such a prediction must rest on a more compelling similarity between our culture, history, legal tradition, and present circumstances than anyone has demonstrated. Without such a demonstration, the argument will not succeed. By stating his argument in this manner, however, Kamisar has led several later commentators to believe that they have refuted the general wedge argument when they have shown that Kamisar's particular type of causal prediction is unsound.[19] To be cogent, however, Kamisar need not have couched his argument as a prediction. For the above comparison to have force, one need not predict that the retarded and the insane will be disposed of; one need only show that the mooted position logically leads to untenable conclusions if fairly applied to all relevantly similar cases. This requirement, that a proposal be fairly applied to all similar cases, is at the core of any system of law or morality. If the essence of law is seen as a system of general rules that define certain classes of acts as beyond what the community can permit, then the very notion of law itself may contain the premise that its rules must apply similarly to similar cases.[20] This principle that Kamisar should have used represents the most basic requirement of justice, one accepted by moralists and statesmen of whatever persuasion: treat similar cases similarly. If any proposal cannot meet such a test of fair application without repugnant results, it must be discarded.

Kamisar should have taken this route; we shall follow it often here. As we shall see, many a proposal to legitimate some form of euthanasia fails this minimal test. Before we can examine cases and proposals, however, we need to test the usefulness of the central distinctions that abound in the euthanasia literature and determine whether or not any of these distinctions help to shape a sound policy for public judgment and practice.

122

Traditional Distinctions in Discourse on Euthanasia

Voluntary / Nonvoluntary

The most obvious distinction found in the literature concerns whether the patient decides that he or she would rather be dead. Is it his or her voluntary choice to die, or has someone else merely decided that it would be best that someone be dead? Miss Quinlan, for example, was incapable of any choice. However caring the motive, however humane the result, others made the choice; she did not.

Some people believe this distinction often has compelling significance. James Rachels suggested in a recent essay that mercy killing be made a legally acceptable justification for killing someone; a defendant could present compelling evidence of the wishes of the deceased, just as one could present a self-defense justification for homicide.[21] This would merely require the defendant to prove the competent consent of the person to being killed. It also assumes the central importance of the distinction between voluntary and nonvoluntary euthanasia.

But Rachels's proposal is a dubious one. And it makes two dubious assumptions:

1. every competent patient's request should be honored;
2. competency can be assessed independently of the reasonableness of the course of action that the agent or one's friend proposes to undertake.

The first assumption is uneventful and widely agreed upon, but the second is not. If competency is regarded as Rachels wishes to—as a threshold beyond which the choice of the patient must be respected—then such abstraction from the actual choice of the patient will not do. It is extremely unlikely that we would wish to honor the choice of someone who wished to be drawn and quartered or who asked to have his or her hands cut off as a means of seeking restitution before God for some sin. I submit that our refusal to honor such requests would have little to do with the mental state of the individual, except insofar as the request itself is regarded as so bizzare as to be seen as evidence for some degree of incompetence. But inspection of this approach shows many difficulties. The consent of the victim has never been allowed to mitigate or absolve a person of a charge of homicide. Active mercy killing of the sick is clearly a species of homicide with nothing of importance to distinguish it from the more common varieties. So, unless we are willing to undertake a profound revision of homicide law, we must conclude, that for legal and policy purposes, consent to active mercy killing is an irrelevant feature, and any distinction based on consent is untenable.

It has been widely assumed, however, that in cases of so-called passive euthanasia, where life-saving treatment is merely withdrawn or withheld, the situation changes. But to be cogent this difference must rest on a willingness to accede to the desires of the patient in every case, even for the most distressed patient. This, of course, seems so unreasonable that few are really prepared to go that far. Absent such a singular commitment, however, we will need to know which choices from which patients need be respected and which not. In short, it seems that we will need to know when it would be reasonable for an individual, in a given situation, to conclude that life really is not worth living. But once we advance a claim to such knowledge, it seems patently unjust to fail to act on such wisdom when confronted with patients who cannot choose or act for themselves.

The common way out of this dilemma is to claim that we can assess whether or not we should accede to the wishes of a patient independently of an evaluation of the reasonableness of what one proposes to do with our help. We shall discuss such a claim later but we may anticipate that discussion briefly at this point. However widely held this maneuver may be it is largely a seductive fiction as far as practice is concerned. It is very difficult to conceive what evidence regarding the incapacities of the patient might be presented at this point other than the quality of the choices one does make, the ends one aims at, and the reasons for which one undertakes them. Someone who wishes to have one's hands cut off as punishment for evil deeds is not, in this society, going to have that wish respected or aided, no matter how normal one's cognitive processes appear in other respects. The choice itself is so outside the boundary of what is even plausibly reasonable that we simply will not respect it; especially we will not aid one in carrying it out.

Properly thought out, therefore, such considerations lead us to conclude that there must be some threshold of reasonableness set forth which can help us assess whether an individual patient's choice is so outside the boundary that we need not honor it. But as we have noted once such a standard is set forth, the theoretical cogency of a distinction between voluntary and nonvoluntary euthanasia disappears.

Active / Passive

For many authors this distinction is quite controversial, if not in fact untenable.[22] For others, it is sound, with an established pedigree in philosophy, law, and public policy.[23] Generally speaking, the distinction refers to whether a physician actively kills the patient in some manner, such as by a lethal injection, or whether a physician simply withdraws or withholds therapies that might save or sustain the life of the patient. It is, as we shall see, difficult to produce any really compelling distinction between these two sorts of activities that would work in law and policy.

Traditionally, neither the individual nor the family could expect the physician to honor a request to kill the patient. At law mercy killing remains homicide for very good reasons. Admitting the propriety of mercy killing will require us to produce a statutory definition of a life not worth living; yet even the most devoted advocates of euthanasia have been incapable of setting forth an acceptable definition. As we saw earlier, this is even true in those cases where the patient can state his or her wishes in these matters. The most compelling cases, however, will surely be those in which the individual cannot state any choice. As a matter of practice, those who are capable of clearly stating their own wishes will usually be in a position to take their own lives without involving family, friends, or physicians. But those who—burdened with illness, weakness, debilitation, or unconsciousness—are unable to take such steps themselves surely present the most difficult cases. But these cases are precisely those in which the capacity of the patient to choose reasonably is most in question.

Karen Quinlan surely provides a good case in point: many commentators would say that her tragic life should be ended as quickly and painlessly as possible. Yet someone else, not Karen, must make the decision that death is in her best interest.

We face, then, this question: is there any cogent distinction—one that can serve as a foundation of public policy—between killing Miss Quinlan and removing the medical apparatus that sustains her life? It seems to me that the cogency of any such general distinction is difficult to maintain. Consider these two cases:

Case I

A person with severe brain damage and paralysis from an auto accident is not dead and is not dying. The patient is alert but brain damage renders him or her clearly incompetent to choose appropriate medical care for himself. The family, believing the life to be worthless, requests the physician to end it painlessly.

Case II

An elderly patient with dementia—rendering him or her incompetent—becomes seriously ill with infection. The family, believing that his or her life is not worth living, requests the physicians to withhold antibiotics, knowing that this will inevitably cause the infection to spread and the patient to die.

These cases are clearly equivalent in all relevant particulars. The end sought in both cases is the same and the means chosen in both instances will be effective in bringing about that end. In both cases the contemplated actions will result in the death of the patient. In assigning responsibility for various wrongs, the *sine qua non* theory of causal responsibility, which is fundamental in law, seems to me to be broadly correct, with some caveats. This action is clearly the crucial *sine qua non* in determining whether the patient lives or dies; therefore, in both cases the physician may be reasonably held to have caused the death of the patient.[24]

Since the means chosen and the consequences produced are equivalent, the only remaining point at which a distinction can be drawn is the intent of the agent. This is the burden of the much discussed principle of the "double effect." An agent may, it is claimed, foresee a consequence of one's behavior for which one is not morally responsible since one intended to produce another simultaneous consequence. For example, the physician may intend to relieve a patient's pain, knowing that a higher dose of medication may also depress the patient's respiration and lead to death. Provided the physician only intends to relieve the patient's pain, he or she would, on this account, not be morally responsible for the death of the patient even if one knew that would be the likely result of one's actions.[25]

When one directly kills the patient, for example, with a lethal injection, one must, it is claimed, intend the result and thus be culpable for it. Whatever good ends are sought by such acts cannot be realized unless the patient is dead; the agent, insofar as he or she wishes to achieve these ends, must intend the death of the patient.

The patient's death is the immediate effect and object of the killing. The beneficent purposes which are often involved in euthanasia decisions cannot be realized unless the person is dead. Thus the pain, suffering, or expense can be ended only if the patient's life is ended. Direct killing necessarily involves the intention of the death of the person being killed.[26] But one can remove or withhold therapy for any of several reasons, some of which may not involve a culpable intent to bring about the death of the person. Thus the principle of the double effect is essentially a claim that the difference in the intent of the agent may ground a moral distinction between acts of removing or withholding medical care and actively killing another human being.

Many objections have been raised to this principle in recent years.[27] Some of these are cogent, others less so. It may be that a sufficiently nuanced and revised version of the principle will be an important part of an adequate moral theory. At least a sua-sive case can be made on its behalf.

But whatever its fate as a part of moral reflection, its utility in law and public policy is deeply problematic. However the principle is revised or amended, the essential claim must be that culpability rests with intent, not with means or conse-quences of behavior. This is admitted by all defenders of any form of the principle.[28] At this point the difficulty for public policy becomes obvious: law is consistently incapable of judg-ing the subjective intent of an agent. This is seen in numerous ways in both civil and criminal law, in governmental regula-tions, and in countless other cases of public policy. In tort law, for example, intent is fundamentally presumed on the basis of behavior and its consequences. "A Person is presumed to in-tend the natural and probable consequences of his acts."[29] The consequences of an act which a reasonable person could foresee are presumed to have been intended by the agent.

Even in criminal law the situation does not change funda-mentally. Though distinctions are made partially on the basis of intent—for example, between the various subclasses of homi-cide—two facts suggest that intent is not the crucial judgment even here. First, the most decisive judgment is the claim that an act has occurred which the state should prevent beforehand if possible or punish afterward. This judgment is made not on the basis of intent but on the basis of the actions of the agent and the consequence of these acts of homicide. Furthermore, even where intent is an issue, the presence or absence of intent is almost always judged on the basis of the actions or statements of the agent at the time. Did one plan to kill the victim? Did one stalk him or her? Did one act in a deliberate manner? Such queries, not one's subjective report of what one intended, are crucial in determining where an accused individual's action lies on the homicide spectrum.[30]

It is difficult to conceive of the law operating on any other basis. Judges and juries cannot read minds. Even psychiatric experts are confused and at odds with one another in these matters. To require such an examination of subjective intent is to emasculate the law as a means of establishing guilt and setting forth appropriate punishment. Consider for example the enormous difficulties posed by an intent requirement in discrimination and voting-rights cases or in conspiracy cases. In voting rights cases such difficulties have led to the abandonment of the intent standard as anything more than presumed from behavior.

But if the investigation of subjective intent is beyond the competence of the law and public policy, it seems clear that a coherent principled distinction between the cases described above simply cannot be sustained in law and policy. A leading moralist seems to tacitly admit this: he admits that passive euthanasia may be as reprehensible as active euthanasia in certain cases. What would decide the matter would be the intent of the agent.[31] But in such cases the law would be impotent to judge and punish reprehensible behavior that led to the death of a human being precisely because it cannot undertake the required examination of subjective intent with any likelihood of success.

More fundamentally, there seems to be little to differentiate these cases when considered according to the jurisprudence of homicide law. The homicide law reflects a fundamental decision against allowing one person to decide that another will not live any more and acting on that choice. Aside from the extreme exigencies of self-defense or the very controversial punishment for capital crimes, we grant an equal minimal right to each life, independently of its status or defects. Such a choice may be disputed; but to dispute it is to dispute the whole rationale for the legal prohibition of homicide as it exists in liberal regimes.

If this proposition of the equal minimal worth of each life is taken as essential in our legal and constitutional framework, the cogency of any general distinction between cases one and two above cannot be sustained. In both cases a third party has made a decision for death over life for the affected patient. In agreeing to the request in either case, the physician can either choose to assent to any such choice or can assert that the choice in question ought to be respected. The first position would entail a more fundamental revision of the law of homicide than anyone has yet proposed. As such, we may set it aside here.

129

The second alternative is no better. The assertion by some-one that he or she knows when the request must be honored is a frank presumption that one knows when the normal con-straints of the law regarding homicide or assisting in suicide ought to apply and when not—that is, when the individual's life is not worth living and so not within the scope of protection afforded by law to all other human life. But for policy purposes this is the crucial claim and the means used to put such a belief into practice is infinitely less important.

What now appears obvious is the fact that both passive and active euthanasia require a judgment that a given human life is not worth living anymore and therefore is not entitled to the same protections as other lives. The Roman Catholic moralists who believed that the Quinlans were justified in their request must admit this conclusion or their position will be hopelessly confused. Miss Quinlan was not in pain and she was patently incapable of suffering. Surely it is not to be maintained that her life is to be ended simply because it is an emotional or financial burden to others. Such a claim would lead to preposterous results if fairly applied. Thus the crucial claim must be that Karen's life is no longer worth living for her.[32] Karen's welfare surely must be the fundamental consideration.

If so, then the requisite judgment regarding lives not worth living looms ever larger in our considerations and the fact that her life is to be ended passively recedes in importance. These are matters to which we shall return below.

Suicide / Homicide

The difficulties we have encountered in establishing per-suasive distinctions between active and passive and voluntary and nonvoluntary euthanasia lead to a crucial set of problems for policy: adequately distinguishing the various forms of eu-thanasia from established categories in law and policy which, it is widely recognized, the state has an inherent right to attempt to prevent and in which intervention is usually right. Those who wish to legalize one or another of the various forms of euthanasia have only two courses open to them unless they wish to mount a wholesale attack on the established restrictions on either suicide or homicide. First, they may show that the activity in question is properly classed but should be permitted as a justified exception to the established prohibitions. Secondly, they may dispute the classification itself. In either case clear lines must be drawn between the prohibited and the permitted activities; we are just beginning to see how difficult that will be.

Active mercy killing is universally admitted to be homicide, most often with the consent of the victim.[33] As such, a case must be made that it constitutes an exception to the justified prohibition of murder. Such an exception must be created in a way not to swallow up the force of the general rule. Limiting oneself to cases where the victim consents is hardly reasonable, given the supposed rationales for mercy killing in the first place. If the patient is permanently incapable of consent it is difficult to see how the alleged humanitarian benefits of killing him or her could be served by keeping this person alive. Those who have defended mercy killing have recognized this point and have generally sought to include incompetent patients in their proposals. To date, however, no such commentator has come close to drafting a mercy killing proposal that would not also logically apply to the chronically insane and the retarded. Logically, we are thus being asked to sanction the possible killing of a million or more human beings. I simply do not know how anyone in this moral, legal, and political tradition could endorse such a proposal.

Passive euthanasia is different. Here most courts and commentators have sought to distinguish this class of cases from suicide.[34] Tom Beauchamp has made the most recent sustained attempt to establish this distinction, but his reason for such an effort seems to be little more than obeisance to the vagaries of contemporary thought.[35] In the end, he cannot provide any such cogent, coherent distinction. He admits that the intention of the patient may be the same in both cases. He also admits that the passivity of the agent will not be sufficient to distinguish it from suicide, where the intention of the agent is the same. Still, he believes that generally it can be said that one who refuses treatment is not the cause of one's death, while the suicide usually is. It seems to me, however, that this is simply the wrong way to put the question. The real question is one of responsibility: who is responsible for the death of this human being? If the question is put in such terms, the answer seems plain—in both cases, the patient is responsible for his or her death. It was plainly within one's capacity to choose either life or death for oneself. One's choice of death is something for which one surely is responsible. One's actions and those of one's physicians are the necessary steps to bringing about one's death; they are the *sine quibus non*. This is the only way in which such cases can be viewed that will square with established precedent in other cases. For example, parent who fails to provide medically necessary life-saving care for his or her child is liable for the child's death. The parent is held responsible for the death of the child, not the bacteria invading the lungs.

Consequently, many moralists have asserted that a proper resolution of these cases need not affect the legal status of suicide intervention by the state of its agents. It is very difficult, however, to maintain this distinction as a general rule. Consider the following two situations:

1. Mr. A is elderly and now confined to a wheelchair. He concludes that life is not worth it and begins refusing to eat. "Life just ain't worth it anymore."

2. Mr. B is elderly and needs to have a leg amputated to save his life. He refuses, saying that if he is confined to a wheelchair, life won't be worth it and he might as well be dead.

It is very difficult to see how any coherent, principled distinction between these two cases can be maintained. In both cases the individual plainly intends to die solely because life itself, in the condition in which he would be forced to live it, is not considered worth it. Neither one is dying; either death can be prevented if the physician or the patient chooses to do so. It is commonly acknowledged, especially in law, that mental health professionals would have a right, perhaps an obligation, to intervene in the first case.

Both patients have clearly set in motion a process that will end in their death. The assertion that patients such as in case two simply wish to "defer to the vagaries of life" or that "It is not they but the natural progress of their ills which will destroy their lives" is simply wrong.[36] It belies that crucial fact that the person has decided to let this happen. Nature has made no such decision for this person. The course that nature will take in these cases is almost wholly at the discretion of the parties involved; they are surely responsible for that course. If true this analysis would drastically affect suicide intervention as well since it can just as easily be claimed that it is not the person but the loss of nourishment that kills the person, when one stops eating for a long period.

It is also difficult to see what relevance various psychiatric theories regarding suicide may have at this point or to find any real help for public policy from such explanations.[37] Whether suicide constitutes "aggression against oneself," as standard psychiatric theory concludes, may or may not be true. Probably, some suicidal persons and some completed suicides can be usefully understood in these terms and others not. It is difficult to conceive of a depressed patient who simply gives up and stops eating in these terms, especially if the term *aggression* is to have anything like its normal meaning. Yet starving oneself in this way is clearly a form of suicide. The point is that public policy and law do not define suicide in terms of psychiatric theory because of the changing nature of these theories and the inability of public decision makers to undertake the extensive psychiatric examinations required. Suicide is defined in terms of behavior and intervention is permitted irrespective of the theoretical perspective within which psychiatrists may understand the behavior.

Finally, it is sometimes claimed that suicide involves a specific intent to die, produced by some active agent employed by the individual for this purpose. On this basis it is claimed that the necessary distinction is obvious. The problems with such a claim as this ought to be obvious by now. It is not at all clear that suicide need involve an active agent. The patient in case

133

one who has stopped eating is every bit as suicidal as the man who wishes to blow his brains out. Intervention with both sorts of acts would be permitted under typical suicide intervention statutes. The problems with an "intent" analysis have been discussed earlier. Subjective intent is impossible to judge in the required manner and objective intent judged from behavior would show the two cases to be equivalent. Even the intent of these two patients may be similar.

The result of our analysis is to render problematic any systematic, coherent differentiation between suicide and the refusal by the patient of clearly life-saving medical therapy. In all those particulars which public judgments can note, the two sets of cases cannot be distinguished in any general fashion. There may be ways in which such a distinction can be made on philosophical or psychiatric grounds in some specific cases but the cogency of these moves is arguable and their usefulness in the formation of policy is dubious.

Separating the actions of the physician in withdrawing medical care from homicide is as difficult as distinguishing the patient's action from suicide. Most writers seem to follow George Fletcher's now well-known attempt to classify this withdrawal as an omission. He argues that, absent a prior relationship between the physician and the patient, such omissions should be governed typically by a Samaritan standard in which the physician may treat the patient if he wishes but is not legally required to do so. He may be a "good Samaritan" and treat but he does not commit homicide if he refuses to do so.[38] Professor Fletcher's description of the cases in which this analysis supposedly works reveals much of his argument and its weaknesses. Suppose, he suggests, a car is parked on a hill without the brakes on. If I, as a passerby, notice this and fail to set the brakes I am surely not legally responsible for the damage that results when the car rolls down the hill. I failed or omitted to perform a certain act, but I am not legally liable for having failed to do so, irrespective of whatever moral blame I must bear.

Unfortunately this analogy is not apposite for the case of

the physician in most situations. The typical patient is not in a completely unrelated position *vis-à-vis* the physician like the stranger in distress or the car parked on the hill whom the physician or the passerby may ignore without fear of liability. Very few decisions not to treat are made when the patient first enters the hospital. As in the case of Karen Quinlan, they are made only after the diagnostic and therapeutic measures of an extensive hospital stay. Only then is the decision made to withhold further attempts at treatment and to withdraw life-sustaining therapy such as respirators, antibiotics and so forth.

Except in special circumstances, when the patient first presents himself to the physician—for example, comes to an emergency room—the physician simply will not know enough about the immediate medical condition of the patient to make a responsible decision about treatment to properly inform the patient. Only after such information is gathered can decisions be made; frequently, such patients will require that life-support measures be undertaken while the information is being gathered. In these ways such decisions are closer to this analogy: suppose a car without brakes is parked on a hill and held in place with a strong rope. I cut the rope and the car rolls down the hill and damages the car and someone's house. It seems clear that I am both legally and morally responsible for the damage to house and to the car, irrespective of whatever relation obtained between me, the owner of the car, or the owner of the house.

The similarity of this case to the situation of Miss Quinlan, tethered to life by a respirator and a feeding tube is obvious. Once the similarity is granted, the attempt to distinguish the withdrawing of medical care from one of the many species of homicide seems to fail at least on these grounds.

Suppose in the above analogy, however, that the only damage was to the car itself. I would still be responsible for the damage. Whether I should be blamed or punished for it would depend on whether the owner pressed charges against me. If the owner saw nothing of value in the car, he or she might not press charges or he or she might actually welcome an opportunity to collect from the insurance company. In short, if I am to be absolved of blame for cutting the rope and causing the damage to the car, it is not because I did not destroy the car but because the car itself was not worth keeping around. The act is excused as an exception because of the worthlessness of the car.

What we shall see more trenchantly below in our review of some court cases is that this precise judgment is impossible to avoid the case of euthanasia. The similarities of these cases to the common sorts of activities that law and policy have proscribed for centuries is obvious. Distinguishing them in ways serviceable as public policy is impossible in a clear coherent manner. What results is the silent assumption that this act is reasonable because the life in question really is not worth living anymore. Like the worn-out car, it is of so little value that the physician who cuts its tether to life is not blameworthy for his act.

Terminal / Nonterminal Patients

Of the available distinctions only one is reasonably coherent and unproblematic enough to be plausibly considered as a matter of law and policy. This is the distinction between those patients who are terminally ill and those who are in some other category such as chronically ill or comatose. For the terminally ill patient, the question of whether he or she lives or dies as a result of disease has already been answered. The patient is going to die. The only question that remains under the control of the patient or the physician is when he or she will die. The physician or the patient may be able to decide whether one dies sooner rather than later but in deciding to withdraw treatment they are not logically required to conclude that the patient would be better off dead. The question is no longer before them.

While this distinction is not as tidy as some commentators suggest, I submit that it is clear enough to be plausibly considered in law and policy.[39] To illuminate its contours, consider the simple act of removing a patient from a respirator. If the patient is not terminally ill then I believe that the only plausible description of the act is to say that one was causally responsible for the death of the patient. One did not merely permit death to occur; an action was the necessary step in bringing about the result. That is, it was the *sine qua non* in the death of the patient and as such this act may be only described as causing the death of the patient. The question at this point is not whether one might persuasively defend one's action, but that on any acceptable view of causation he or she must be described as causing the death of the patient.

On the other hand it is not at all clear that the physician's activities can be described in the same terms if the patient is terminally ill. At the very least it seems to me that we can no longer described the physician's action in the *sine qua non* framework of causation and moral responsibility that is fundamental in law. The patient here will die anyway and the actions of the doctor will have no effect in this regard. It therefore seems to me at least plausible to conclude that the doctor is not causally responsible for the death of the patient.

More significantly, there are important policy reasons to prefer this distinction. For the terminal patient, neither the agent nor the law need be concerned with the hopelessly elusive question of a life not worth living. It is enough merely to say that an individual need not prolong the process of dying. Moving beyond this to include the chronically ill, the debilitated, and the comatose will inevitably entail insoluble problems setting forth a proper rule or the abdication of any prohibition of suicide or assisting in suicide when the individual or the family concludes that life is not worth it.

Most current living-will legislation limits itself to cases of the terminally ill. In the typical legislation, a terminally ill patient is empowered to sign a written document that instructs one's physicians to remove specified forms of care, even if one should become incompetent to make such a request oneself. In keeping with the context of such cases, the legislation goes as far as it can without calling into question convictions about the worth of individual human lives that lie at the foundation of our polity and which are embodied in centuries of common law development.

The Life Not Worth Living

Theory

It now appears clear that the question of what constitutes a life not worth living cannot be avoided in any of the commonly accepted subspecies of euthanasia. Except where the patient is actually terminally ill, any reasonable version of a euthanasia policy in any of its subspecies seems to require some criteria in terms of which those involved may reasonably conclude that the person does not have a life worth living. Without such criteria no policy can be sustained.

This conclusion is most obviously true in those cases involving incompetent patients. It is sheer fiction to believe that anything else is going on in these cases than a decision by the family and or the physician that this life is not worth living. The individual is making no such choice. By definition the patient can make no choice. Absent the rare case where compelling evidence of one's desires is presented, such as a written document, one's liberty to choose one's medical care cannot possibly be a relevant consideration. It is plain nonsense to assert otherwise, though some courts have done so in recent decisions.[40] The patient in these cases simply cannot exercise any personal right for oneself; the family must do so, that is, they must make the decision. This, however, is not the patient's exercise of a right at all. For example, does it make any sense to say that a severely retarded person is exercising a first amendment right when his or her family takes him or her to church or that one's right to know about public matters is exercised by being placed in front of a television set while the news is on, when one cannot understand eighty per cent of the words being used? The answers to these queries seem obvious, as does the analogy to the euthanasia case.

Moreover families do not usually enjoy absolute power over the lives and fortunes of those in their care. This is exactly the import of the right to die cases themselves. Families like the Quinlans sought authority which it was not at all clear that they had. For example, if a family wished to undertake a religious fast for a week, they would certainly have a constitutionally protected right to do so. However, if they also made a pro-foundly retarded child fast, they would certainly be abusing the child by depriving the child of needed food for reasons he or she could never understand and which would be of no benefit to him or her. At that point the child is exercising no religious right; those who would require the fast, like the zealot who refuses blood transfusions for a critically ill child, makes a decision with little constitutional standing.

In all such cases the hidden premise is the belief that it is in fact reasonable that a patient dies. What justifies the Quinlans in their act, if anything, is the belief that what they propose is in their daughter's best interest. She would be better off dead. Claims by courts and commentators concerning her right to refuse treatment are an attempt to evade the implications of this central question.

It is often argued that a direct confrontation with quality of life criteria may be avoided in many of the most compelling cases through two alternative moves employed with different classes of patients. For the patient who asks for the removal of life-sustaining therapy or to be killed, it is often claimed that we should only concern ourselves with the competency of the patient to choose, not the content of the choice thus made.[41] On the other hand, it is claimed that comatose patients are not persons, and therefore are not bearers of a serious right to life that must be overridden by quality of life considerations.

Initially, the competency claim in particular seems plausible. It has, however, serious flaws. Any assessment of whether we must respect a given choice will certainly entail an investigation of the reasons given for the choice. For example, consider a patient who says "stop all treatment because Martians are coming to cure me with light rays." Clearly we would not honor his or her request even if, objectively, we might be comfortable with a patient refusing the treatment this patient wants stopped. The patient's reason is so outside the bounds of what is reasonable that it simply does not provide adequate grounds for removing life-sustaining medical care.

Similarly a patient who asks a physician to amputate a perfectly healthy limb as a punishment for sin is hardly likely to have such a request fulfilled. If a person wishes to be maimed in some permanent way, I believe we would normally require very strong reasons for such an action before we would assist him or her in any way. What he or she aims at is, *prima facie,* so unreasonable that it, *ipso facto,* arouses strong suspicions that no such reasons can be given.

Usually, patients do not request the physician or family to take a course of action that will end in their death. Such a request is obviously out of the ordinary. What would make it reasonable is a plausible belief that whatever life the patient would have after therapy would not be worth living. Thus, it seems clear that at least the reasons offered by the patient must be assessed by those whom the patient wishes to assist in carrying out such requests. In the cases at hand, this will require an assessment of the claim that life in one's condition is not worth living. Unless we wish to abdicate all responsibility for a conscientious judgment, we must decide that it is utterly implausible for the individual to reach the required conclusion about the life one must live. It appears, therefore, that we need to produce an acceptable definition of when it would be within the bounds of reason for a patient, family, or physician to conclude that this life is not worth it.

The fundamental problem with the competency maneuver in these cases is its assumption that the distinction between competency and incompetence is the crucial judgment in the justification of medical paternalism. In the standard account of paternalism, the necessary and sufficient conditions for paternalistic interventions by physicians are:

1. the incompetence of the patient and
2. the benefits of the proposed action.

If the patient is incompetent and the action is medically in the best interest of the patient then the physician may act.[42]

Though a full analysis of this account is beyond the scope of my discussion here, it is far too simple. Two points may be noted in this regard. First, it may be that on any plausible account of rationality a particular patient holds utterly irrational beliefs about his or her disease. Yet, we would find paternalistic interventions bad as a policy. Hence, we permit the patient to act in ways equivalent to cases of actual declared incompetence. One person may hear the voice of spacemen telling one to refuse treatment and another may hear the voice of god in a religious text or a private spiritual experience. The former will almost certainly have his or her competency questioned and persistence in this belief may very well lead to a judgment of incompetence. Nothing similar is likely to befall the religious believer, even though the claim seems epistemically equivalent.

The difference in treatment is not triggered by the cases but by the policy implications of paternalism in these instances. A policy that permitted intervention in the irrational activities of religious believers would strike far too deeply at the presumption of competency in otherwise normal adults. Far too many adults are involved in religious communities that require acts that make no sense in any human terms, to make paternalism acceptable as a policy in such medical cases.[43]

Secondly, the standard account overlooks the countervailing importance of individual liberty in these cases. It may be that strictly speaking the physician cannot avoid an assessment of the reasonableness of what the individual proposes to do, even in the refusal of treatment cases. However, we might still conclude that the importance of individual liberty requires that in most of these cases the person ought to be permitted to do as one wishes, simply as a result of a balance between the competing moral claims of the worth of life and individual liberty and the onerous and probably unsuccessful implications of intervention. That is, in most cases of otherwise normal and fully informed adults we must restrain the impulse to intervene because of the importance of individual liberty that our society nourishes and values.

As the above discussion noted, what typically occurs in these cases is that this countervailing interest in liberty is smuggled into the discussion of competency. Competency assessments are not neutral. They require the assessment of the choices people make, even the medical choice at hand. In cases involving otherwise normal adults who propose to refuse therapy, we typically permit the interest in liberty to be decisive, except where more assistance, and therefore agreement, is required by others. If you ask me to be involved in your case, then I must judge what you propose to do and my role in it. If it is something I am morally prohibited from doing, such as giving you poison, then the community as a whole must agree to my involvement in law or policy. But if all that you ask me to do is permit you to undertake some act, then I must first ask what the costs in loss of liberty to you are if I intervene.

The claim that comatose individuals are not persons, or, alternatively, are not bearers of a right to life, is more problematic than claims regarding competency.[44] Many arguments are alleged in defense of this view; two of these are central and widely employed. The first trades on the emerging consensus regarding "brain death." It is argued that the very concept of brain death necessarily entails a distinction between a human being as a biological entity and the consciousness of self and world that is the characteristic of a person and which requires cerebral functioning at levels higher than the brainstem that is necessary for the maintenance of biological life. What we have done, it is said, is to express our belief that the human being *qua* biological entity is not valuable enough to merit normal rights and protections in the evasive language of *brain death*. Honesty, it is asserted, ought to compel awareness of this fiction and a consistent adherence to the distinction between "human being" and "person" that it entails. Thus, rather than asserting that the comatose patient has a low quality of life, we might simply say that he or she has no personeity which is the basis of rights and protections.[45]

But this maneuver is successful only if we can plausibly maintain an equivalence between the comatose patient and the brain-dead patient. It is a biological fact that the comatose patient has a continuously functioning physiological system, so equivalence will not be found in that manner. Perhaps we could say that in both cases the patient is alive but lacking in some value that is necessary as a condition of being treated as a full person with rights to life and other human goods.

At this point however a crucial difference seems to appear, one that is signaled by clinical signs. Patients who are brain dead by the current whole-brain standard cannot be kept alive mechanically for more than a very short time. In almost all cases they will have irreversible cardiac arrest within a week. Moreover, these patients have all of the usual clinical signs of death. They are motionless, incapable of reflexes, unresponsive even to painful stimuli, and have fixed pupils. The whole process of autoregulation of body physiology once performed by the brain is now gone. Patients with irreversible coma, on the other hand, still are responsive to stimuli, still can track light with their eyes, maintain temperature and blood pressure, metabolize food and oxygen. The brain's central biological function of regulating the physiological equilibrium of the body is still intact.[46]

The central role of the brain in the existence of a human being is thus its capacity to integrate the various organ systems and physiological processes into a functioning whole and to regulate these various systems so that the equilibrium necessary for life is maintained. Without this integration and regulation, life cannot be sustained. But this necessary function cannot be transferred to a mechanical substitute as the functions of some individual organs can. Thus it can be cogently argued that the one essential characteristic of the existence of human being as a biological entity is the existence of a functioning brainstem sufficient to perform the necessary integrating function.

If death is seen as a biological point, then it makes very good sense to identify that point in human life with irreversible cessation of all brain function, not with the absence of higher brain functions. In fact, higher-brain formulations of the brain-death concept are usually patently moral in their import: they identify something of value in human beings and conclude that, once this quality is irreversibly gone, then one ought to be treated as if one lacks the rights normally accorded persons in our moral order. But this is a moral argument, not a deduction from a set of biological facts, nor from a reasonable concept of death based on and explaining those facts.

Perhaps the strongest claims made in this regard are those which say straightforwardly that the comatose, and perhaps,

143

the senile, the retarded, and other classes of human beings lack essential attributes of persons and hence bear only socially ascribed rights based on a utilitarian calculation that such an ascription is required to produce a caring, compassionate, moral community which best serves the interests of persons proper. For the comatose, however, it is said that we can set aside this fiction if the communal order it sustains will not be seriously weakened.[47]

Though this distinction between "human being" and "person" forms no part of the common law, it has a certain attractiveness of its own. Nevertheless, it is both deeply flawed and incapable of avoiding the concept of a life not worth living. The most crucial flaw in the strongest version of this maneuver is the confusion between the preconditions for moral agency and the preconditions for being a bearer of any rights at all. Given the distinction between human being and person, it is a truism that moral agency and hence obligations can only be ascribed to persons. But to extend this argument as a precondition of rights in more than the extended, utilitarian sense noted above, is doubtful. The claim seems to be that the very concept of morality requires that we treat persons with respect for their autonomy, that is, respect them as ends, not means, in Kant's sense. This is supposedly the ground of a strong sense of personal rights which are a necessary part of the fabric of a moral community of persons. In other words, respect for persons is the basis of a moral community within which reciprocal rights and obligations emerge to sustain and protect this respect. But the very concept of such respect presupposes the existence of persons as moral agents.

Unfortunately, this argument is incapable of sustaining much of the cogency of our fundamental concepts regarding rights. Rights are not unlimited. We do not believe that, in general, interference with any of our activities involves the violation of some serious rights. If I am prevented from swimming because the city has closed its pools in a budget crisis, my rights have surely not been violated. But if I am threatened with severe punishment because I have more than two children, it surely seems part of our moral universe to claim that my rights are being violated. It is precisely such differentiation among acts and the ends toward which they aim that the respect-for-persons formulation of the basis of rights misses. The very limitations inherent in the concept of rights points to the view that some human endeavors are held to be of such moral import that very special reasons must be adduced for any interference with them. However, the respect for persons formulation cannot sustain such a distinction. Going to the park or bearing children are equal in this respect: both are autonomous choices of a free moral agent. Since the very concept of rights seems to entail a differentiation such as that noted above, rights themselves must be based on a moral understanding that is prior to and more fundamental than respect for persons as autonomous moral agents.

Furthermore, while clearly personhood in this strong sense is required for moral agency, and hence for the exercise of some rights, for example, the right to practice a religion of one's choice, it is not at all clear that the possession and exercise of all rights require personhood in this sense. To say that I have a right to X is, in the first instance, to say something about what you may not do, not what I may or may not do. Where it is a question of my right to conduct some activity, surely I must be capable of the required performance. But if it is a question of already possessing some good, then the necessity of a capacity for moral agency or personhood appears less obvious. A retarded person with a large inheritance has a right to his or her inheritance, irrespective of how it is used or who uses it on his or her behalf; a serious wrong would be committed by my stealing it. Similarly, I submit that to be a bearer of a right to life, I only need be in possession of that great good, that is, I only need be alive. There is no reason to suppose that I need to be a person in the strong sense to have the right to life on exactly the same terms as anyone else.

Even a weaker claim that rights presuppose the having of interests which are necessarily not had by the comatose patient is in trouble here.[48] Individuals surely have rights regarding things in which they have no interests. A confirmed bachelor still has a right to beget children and I may not sterilize him at my whim. Nor can it be held that the conscious awareness of the right or interest is necessary else any concept of rights held by the senile or the retarded will be difficult to sustain. It therefore seems that any necessary connection between having interests or being conscious of interests or rights and actually having such rights must be denied.

Even more to the point of our current discussion is the patent fact that none these moves avoids a quality of life judgment on the lives of some patients. If we may withhold care or even kill when such treatment will not adversely affect the moral order then we need to know when this point is reached. Surely if it is reached in the case of normal children, who are not persons,[49] then we need to know when it is reached, that is, how close to or far from the norm need one be before one cannot be killed with impunity. But this is simply another way of asking when it is that whatever worth is attached to individual lives is so diminished as to be overridden by such negative factors as pain, suffering, physical handicaps, or cognitive incapacities.

Criteria

When we turn to examine the proffered criteria for such an assessment we are prepared from our assessment of the infanticide literature for the vagueness, confusions, and contradictions that appear frequently. For example, in a pair of spirited defenses of active mercy killing for both competent and incompetent patients, Professor Arval Morris has argued that the patients who could be killed either on their own consent or the consent of others when they are incompetent are those who are in an "irremediable condition."[50] The required irremediable condition is further defined thus:

> "Irremediable condition" means either (1) a serious physical illness which is diagnosed as incurable and terminal and which is expected to cause a person severe distress or to render him incapable of a rational existence or (2) a condition of brain damage or deterioration such that a person's normal mental faculties are severely and irreparably

impaired to such an extent that he has been rendered incapable of leading a rational existence.[51]

As a proposed statute this is astonishingly poor. Nowhere is the key concept "rational existence" defined with any precision. No clear lines are drawn to mark off acceptable from unacceptable behavior. No criteria are offered for those who will have to implement such a law. Nothing is offered here except vague claims about the lack of a rational existence and the suffering such a life involves. How physicians are to make such a choice is never mentioned nor is the more important question of why they should make it at all explored.

The problem is that modern political philosophy and jurisprudence have systematically excluded these questions from public life. They may be discussed publicly, but only as matters of personal preference or religious opinion—not as matters of law or public choice. Morris, however, wishes to adopt some public standard, a rational existence, as the *sub rosa* qualification to the presumed equal minimal worth of each human life. Instead of all men being endowed with such a right to life, we now have all men not determined by a couple of doctors to be incapable of a rational existence. In this sense Morris takes a path that the founders of liberalism specifically rejected.

This fundamental departure from our political and legal tradition has serious implications. Lacking any public agreement on the matter of a rational existence, citizens are left to their own resources of religious opinion, personal experience, and even prejudice. Such a state of affairs leads directly to the most pervasive and central injustice possible in a liberal regime—the refusal to treat similar cases similarly. If, under this policy, one set of physicians decides one way and another set decides another way in a similar case, how can that even be minimally fair? Morris seems oblivious to the facts of human experience and empirical data that suggest such variance is almost certain to occur under his law, and he offers us no way to avoid it or even minimize its effects.[52] Furthermore, Morris's standard logically includes hundreds of thousands of retarded and chronically insane persons who are demonstrably incapable of a rational existence under any plausible definition of that term. This result is, perhaps, the most telling objection to such proposals. It represents so momentous a departure from our moral, legal, and political tradition that I simply do not see how one can endorse it.

These recommendations represent the confusion and contradictions one finds in much of the literature on the right to die. Some writers offer no standard at all, merely a series of cases in which they believe either active or passive euthanasia is justified.[53] This may be acceptable in a discussion of moral issues or as a means of raising the question for discussion but it simply will not do as an answer to serious questions of public policy. If these authors wish us to provide in law and policy exceptions to or revisions of long established principles and the rights they enshrine, then they must tell us how wide these exceptions will be. Until they do, in terms that still preserve the force of the general rule, they offer nothing of real use to those actually charged with shaping public standards and practices.

Professor Morris is hardly the only author who presents standards for moral choice or policy making that are vague, contradictory, and ill conceived. Terms like *burden, hardship, suffer* abound, though the various authors give few clear definitions in the literature. For example, one recent author claims that nonvoluntary euthanasia of the permanently comatose is morally right. To substantiate her claim she argues that it can be in the best interests of such people to be dead rather than exist as they must. And there the argument ends. The rest of the case being made is deduced from naked assertions about the terrible affliction of the patient and hidden assumptions about how the patient faces an empty life or one filled with suffering. Of course, none of these terms is precisely defined nor is the key concept of "best interest" ever delineated with sufficient precision to make it useful for practice. Since the comatose patient is incapable of suffering and is not in pain, one wonders what makes his or her life so terrible. Moreover, how are we to know that the life is empty? To say that euthanasia is acceptable in these cases in any form requires clear precise answers to these questions. Without them, the whole case collapses.[54]

Other authors simply state that the right to die is part of the meaning of the right to privacy and should therefore receive constitutional protection in every case and in every form. Some offer reasons or, more frequently, assertions about when euthanasia would be acceptable; but then they offer statutes that provide for euthanasia whenever anyone wants it. These are the far end of the current discussion; they simply ignore the fundamental constitutive core of liberal regimes that is founded on the concept of inalienable rights and equal worth.[55] More common are those who do provide some idea of when life is not worth living but whose articulation of this crucial point is so confused that it provides little guidance for public or professional practice.[56]

Mercy Killing: Making It Legal

In the last two years, the question of mercy killing and assisting in suicide has emerged in a serious and unexpected way in the current discussion about care for the terminally ill and gravely debilitated. A major national organization, the Hemlock Society, has moved beyond the position of other similar organizations and has actively pressed for the repeal of all laws prohibiting assisting in suicide and mercy killing with the consent of the patient.[57] National news programs have made this topic a matter of scrutiny and court cases with widely disparate outcomes have made it a serious issue for law and public policy.[58]

Though any such change would be a momentous reversal of centuries of common law development, it cannot be dismissed for that reason alone. Novelty is not always imprudent. It is however, here, extremely unwise and ill conceived. The proponents of this change seem to regard it as a simple extension of the acknowledged right of self-determination that all competent patients have. On this view, the person who kills me at my request is simply the instrument of my death. For example, suppose I rig a timing device to fire a gun at a certain spot in five minutes, giving me time to return and lie in that spot. The machine is part of the causal chain that will lead to my death but it is set in motion by the free decision that I surely have a right to make for myself. But, the argument runs, this example is still sound if another person pulls the trigger instead of a timing device. It is still my decision, deriving from my view of the human good and protected by the same view of individual rights that condemns the forced use of dialysis in otherwise competent patients.

The fundamental weakness in this argument, however, is the way in which this analogy implies that the agent who kills me is nothing more than a robot at my command. The machine certainly can only do what I have set it up to do: shoot at a certain spot at a certain time. It cannot deliberate about whether it ought to comply. It can only do it. At this point the requisite analogy breaks down completely. For one of the most fundamental experiences of human moral agency, especially in cases such as this, is the experience of deliberation, of trying to decide whether I ought to do what someone has asked me to do. Even when you can command me to do it, I must still deliberate, I must decide that the arguments you offer for the act or the rewards or punishments that you can bestow are sufficient grounds for my doing as you wish.

But if the mercy killer must deliberate about his action, then clearly the fact of your request does not, by itself, constitute sufficient grounds for compliance with your request. What one needs is some independent ground for believing that compliance is reasonable. One must have some plausible reason for doing what one is normally prohibited from doing, killing another human being.

Furthermore, the mercy killer is not being asked to merely stop interfering in the life of the patient, with elaborate medical technology or drug injections that he does not want. He is asking me to assist him in doing what he wants done. He does not simply want me to stop restraining him from robbing a store, he wants me to hold the gun on the storekeeper while he takes the money. Surely my complicity in such acts requires my believing that what he wishes to do is a reasonable course of action. I do not need to know that it is the best course of action or that it is my preferred course, simply that it is morally acceptable. Even framed in this manner, though, the requisite judgment is extremely significant. Clearly, the mercy killer must make an independent judgment that it is reasonable for someone in this condition to believe that death is better than life. But this puts mercy killing squarely back in the "life not worth living" game, a game for which no one has been able to provide adequate rules. Moreover, any such judgment ought to apply to the competent and the incompetent alike. If the mercy killer on request knows when it would be reasonable for him to kill the competent, he surely must know when to kill the incompetent as well. Clearly, permanently incompetent patients, such as those with advanced Alzheimer's disease, are worse off in human functioning than those whose request supposedly should be honored. At this point, the logical implications of mercy killing have led us directly to a public policy of selective euthanasia that can neither be given a rational terminus nor squared with our most fundamental traditions as a community. In its essential respects, therefore, mercy killing on request cannot avoid the severe difficulties of such policies that we have noted throughout this and previous chapters.

Court Cases—Studies in Confusion

The confusions seen in the various attempts to develop public policy regarding the right to die, especially the attempts to answer the central questions regarding the nature of a life not worth living are mirrored in many recent court decisions dealing with the right to die. Here we can only examine three of the most important sets of cases as examples of the confusions which abound.

Quinlan

The earliest of the recent major decisions was New Jersey's celebrated Quinlan decision, the facts of which we have noted earlier. Here the New Jersey Supreme Court held that the Quinlans had the right to remove life sustaining medical care from their adult comatose daughter.[59] To reach its conclusion the court took recourse in the concept of individual autonomy, which it incorrectly designated as a privacy right. As noted before,[60] this maneuver is sheer fiction. It is not Karen's autonomous choice that is at stake; what is at stake is what is best for her, a fact which the court seems to admit very obliquely.[61] By framing its inquiry in these terms, however, the court masks its most crucial claim—that Miss Quinlan's life should be ended because it is worthless. It attempts to attribute such a choice to Karen herself but even the court admits it has no basis for doing so.[62] No one knows what Karen would want; even her parents could not persuasively make such a claim.

Thus the judgment that Karen's life was not worth living becomes central in two ways. First, it was an essential feature of the best interest test that is the only coherent fashion in which to frame the questions faced by the court and her parents. Secondly, it was the only way in which the court could distinguish its decision in this case from earlier precedents in which it did order life-saving therapy for incompetent patients.

In the other case this very court ordered blood transfusions for a comatose woman whose religious beliefs forbade it. These beliefs were interpreted to the physicians and the court by her mother and friends and were uncontested. The court, however, relying on centuries of common law precedent, found the state's interest in the preservation of life and the prevention of suicide sufficient to order the transfusion.[63] In the *Quinlan* case, the court did not overturn this precedent. Rather, it distinguished these cases in precisely the terms that are our concern here:

> We have no doubt, in these unhappy circumstances, that if Karen were herself lucid for an interval (not altering the existing prognosis of the condition to which she would soon return) and perceptive of her irreversible condition, she could effectively decide to discontinue the life-support apparatus, even if it meant the prospect of natural death. To this extent we distinguish *Heston*, which concerned a severely injured young woman [Dolores Heston], whose life depended on surgery and blood transfusion; who was in such extreme shock that she was unable to express an informed choice [although the court apparently considered

> the case as if the patient's own religious decision to resist
> transfusion were at stake], but most importantly a patient
> apparently salvable to long life and vibrant health;—a situ-
> ation not at all like the present case.
> We have no hesitancy in deciding in the instant diametri-
> cally opposite case that no external compelling interest of
> the state could compel Karen to endure the unendurable,
> only to vegetate a few measurable months with no realistic
> possibility of returning to any semblance of cognitive or
> sapient life.[64]

The plain import of this passage is unmistakable. Miss Heston's life is saved, even against her religious convictions, because her life is worth living. Miss Quinlan's life is to be ended, not because her religious convictions dictate or approve it but simply because the court believed that her life was not worth living anymore. The implication of the court's position is clear. If Karen had a chance to regain sentience, there would have been no deference to the wishes of her parents and quite probably to any statements made by Karen herself, if *Heston* stands. The court simply used whatever right could be conceived of as vaguely applicable in the search for a legal rationale for what it believed was morally best—the release of Karen from what the court termed *unendurable* existence.

Unfortunately, the *Quinlan* court gave little coherent guidance in this uncharted area. It obviously believed that Karen's life is awful, but offered us no idea of how awful a human life must be before it reaches the threshold of unendurability where someone else may be empowered to remove the medical measures sustaining it. Seeking to draw on the established doctrine of substituted judgment, it attempted to attribute desires to Karen that it has absolutely no basis for, except its own assertion that this is what a reasonable person would want.[65] In its attempt to buttress its decision with recourse to the concept of privacy, it was forced to note the intrusiveness of the medical procedure, but gave us no guidance on how intrusive a medical procedure must be before it becomes a matter of privacy.

In the instant case, Mr. Quinlan sought removal of the respirator. He did not seek removal of the feeding tube that provided nourishment to his daughter. Would this fall in the same category of intrusiveness? Any reasonable analysis of the procedures themselves would be hard pressed not to reach such a conclusion. Both the respirator and the feeding tube involve permanent technological intrusion into the body to provide for necessary function that the body cannot now perform: intake of air and food. The two are strikingly similar in this regard, for the gastro-intestinal tract can still process what is taken in and the lungs can still extract oxygen in a form usable by the body. In short the court has given us no guidance on most of the crucial issues at stake.

Saikewicz and Spring

Among the most controversial cases regarding the right to die are those from Massachusetts, chiefly the cases of *Saikewicz* and *Spring*.[66] In *Saikewicz* the patient was a sixty-seven-year-old profoundly retarded man who developed a form of leukemia. Since he had been cared for all his life in an institution, the staff sought the guidance of the court in making decisions regarding his care. The court appointed a guardian *ad litem*; after a hearing it concluded that chemotherapy for leukemia could be withheld. On appeal this judgment was upheld by the highest court in the state.

The court followed the *Quinlan* decision in asserting that were Saikewicz competent, his right of privacy would mean that he could refuse any treatment whatsoever on any grounds, absent serious countervailing claim. It found no such claims to be persuasive in this case and therefore held that Saikewicz would have a right to refuse any medical care. Given Saikewicz's inability to exercise any such right, the court must grant someone else the power to exercise it for him. This is, of course, the same sort of fictitious maneuver we have seen in *Quinlan*. Saikewicz had never been competent, had never chosen any life-plan from which we might gain some insight into what he would want. Furthermore, the court specifically noted that among normal individuals faced with Saikewicz's condition, a majority choose chemotherapy.[67] The only way the court could surmount this fact was by giving up the search for what

Saikewicz would want, or what a rational man would choose, and thereby giving up any attempt to base the decision on his right to decide what is best for him.

After assuming the power to make this decision for Saikewicz, the court concluded that he should not be given chemotherapy, knowing that failure to provide the therapy inevitably meant the death of Saikewicz. In reaching this conclusion, the court considered several factors that may be important in making such a decision. It concluded that two sets of factors are crucial. First, Saikewicz's retardation meant that he would suffer the side effects of therapy without any redeeming understanding of what was happening to him.

> Patients who request treatment know the risks involved and can appreciate the painful side effects when they arrive. They know the reason for the pain and their hope makes it tolerable. To make a worthwhile comparison, one would have to ask whether a majority of people would choose chemotherapy if they were told merely that something outside of their previous experience was going to be done to them, that this something would cause them pain and discomfort, that they would be removed to strange surroundings and possibly restrained for a long time, and that the advantages of this course of action were measured by concepts of time and mortality beyond their ability to comprehend.[68]

In making this maneuver the court departed from its own announced goal of excluding the quality of life of the person from consideration in rendering a decision. By making his suffering under treatment crucial, the court plainly suggested that Saikewicz's life would be more miserable than would the lives of the majority who it admits would choose therapy. It is this very misery that justifies the court in choosing for him a course of action that it believes others would not choose.

The court was led to this conclusion by the way it framed the case. In adopting an expansive view of the right that is to be accorded to Saikewicz, the court was prevented from concluding that he would refuse the treatment because it would not actually save his life, merely prolong his dying, or that it cannot definitely save his life. Either of these is arguably a sound conclusion from the facts as presented, but the court plainly wished no such restriction on the right in question. They wished a broader right to refuse any therapy at all, even where it was a real matter of saving life. In so doing they must conclude as they do, or else choose therapy for Saikewicz.

In a curious way the position of the court is coherent at this point. Since it has excluded a decision based on Saikewicz's grim prognosis and endorsed the broad right of any patient to refuse any therapy, it must also endorse the quality of life decision that such a standard entails. Wishing to extend this right to the incompetent patient, the court is surely not wrong, on its own terms, in using these frank quality of life considerations to determine what it chooses for the patient, without any indication of what the incompetent patient would want.

We shall shortly see the lengths to which this court is prepared to go in endorsing a quality of life standard in the *Spring* decision, in which the court had to override the last competently expressed wish of the patient to adopt a quality of life outcome that it obviously believed to be best. Of course, the broader policy question of allowing third parties to make choices for death when a majority of competent persons faced with analogous choices would not so choose, merely because the third party asserts the misery of the incompetent's life is never discussed. Nor is the logical extension of such a policy to hundreds of thousands of persons like Saikewicz, afflicted with ills from appendicitis to bowel incontinence, ever mentioned.

Viewed broadly, however, the *Saikewicz* decision is confusing. The only way that the decision can be salvaged is by adopting the very conclusion that the court says it wants to avoid: that Saikewicz should not be treated because his life is not worth living. This conclusion and the immense difficulties it raises become more evident in the Massachusetts cases that appeared in the aftermath of the *Saikewicz* decision.

For our purposes one of these cases is crucial, that of Earle Spring.[69] Spring was an eighty-seven-year-old man suffering from chronic organic brain syndrome and end-stage renal disease. The family sought permission from the court to withhold further renal dialysis, with the inevitable result of the death of the patient.

In finding for the family, the court had no clear, competently expressed statement of the patient's wishes to guide it. The nearest thing to such a statement, the patient's desire to stay on dialysis before he became incompetent, clearly cut against the court's decision. Nevertheless, the court concluded that the belief of his wife of fifty-five years as to what he would want must be accorded great weight. However, the court still seemed confused on the crucial question of whether the proposed treatments represented a chance to save a life or merely an opportunity to prolong an already inevitable dying process. In the present case, as in the *Saikewicz* case, there was no dispute as to the patient's lack of competence. In each case the patient was clearly alive and conscious, and suffering from an incurably fatal disease. The treatments in question were intrusive and were life-prolonging rather than life-saving; there was no prospect of cure, or even of recovery of competence. In the *Saikewicz* case, the life-prolonging treatment had not yet begun, and there was urgency with regard to taking action to begin treatment; in the present case the temporary continuation of treatment did not greatly change the situation.[70]

This is confusing. The fact that there is no prospect of cure may not be relevant. Patients with pacemakers are not cured but their lives are indefinitely prolonged and they usually do not die of the disease for which the pacemaker was inserted. If the intrusiveness of the therapy is central then, at a minimum, the court ought to spell out what it means by the use of this term: employing it in the cases of *Saikewicz* and *Spring* is *prima facie* inconsistent.

The hidden assumption here is that, since Mr. Spring has lost the use of his conscious mental faculties, it is reasonable to refuse further therapy, an act that will almost certainly lead to his death. This is what the court knows but will not acknowledge. In order to reach its position, the court must disregard the man's last expressed choice regarding his medical care, specifically the therapy that the court now permits to be removed. As noted above the life-prolonging nature of the treatment cannot be determinative as a moments reflection on the case of a diabetic retarded person will show. Rather, the court must conclude that Mrs. Spring is right: her husband ought to die.[71]

Eichner

The next case we shall examine is that of Brother Fox, the eighty-seven-year-old member of a Catholic religious order who suffered massive brain damage and coma following cardiac arrest during surgery. Unlike the previous cases, which are far more typical, here there was clear evidence of what Brother Fox would want. He had discussed this sort of situation extensively with his religious family and had made clear his wish for no life-sustaining measures in the event he became comatose. The various courts that considered this case might have ended their inquiries at this point, noting the serious respect for individual choice inherent in our political and legal traditions. By not doing so, these courts stepped boldly into the same problems that plagued other courts in the sorts of cases we have just noted.

To begin with, the trial court wisely rejected the notion found in *Quinlan* and *Saikewicz* that any constitutional right of privacy was involved here. They quite properly noted that the privacy right was so ambiguous that it could mean anything one wanted it to and, as usually understood, was most ill suited to cover the case at hand.

> The resolution of the awesome question posed by this case, literally one of life and death for Brother Fox, may hereafter profoundly affect all citizens of this State. No one can foresee the nature of future petitions seeking to apply the conclusion reached here. This consideration also underlines this Court's determination not to base a conclusion on the claim of a right of privacy that is insufficiently defined but nevertheless so attractively worded as to invite unrestrained applications made in its name.[72]

Since privacy was not involved, the trial court turned to common law principles of self-determination found in tort and

158

contract law. Such a right of self-determination, including a right to refuse medical care, may be overridden only in special circumstances. The court specifically noted three such:

1. the protection of minor children from abandonment or trauma,
2. a proper respect for the necessity for physicians to discharge their ethical obligations, and
3. the preservation of human life.[73]

Given the facts of the case, only the third of these considerations was at issue. In resolving it, however, the trial and appellate courts were confused. In their confusion they slid into treacherous waters. At the outset the trial court acknowledged a distinction between those cases in which life can be saved and those where it cannot.[74] In so doing it sought to avoid a fundamental decision regarding the right to intervene in cases where the patient's life can be saved. Unfortunately, the facts of the case will not submit to this analysis. Brother Fox was not dead and he may not have been dying. At the very least he was not dying in the manner we have traditionally considered that a patient is terminally ill from a specific disease like lung cancer. He was, like Miss Quinlan, in a permanent vegetative state with no realistic hope of regaining cognitive function. If he were actually dying, the court's position would be tenable. But he was not. As the court tacitly acknowledged, he is in a hopeless condition with respect to his mental faculties, not his life. If left the respirator there is no way to know if or when this man will die. He could die quickly as most patients do or he could linger for years as did Miss Quinlan.

The partially hidden truth is that the only way to salvage Eichner, on the court's terms, was to conclude that Brother Fox's condition was worthless, not hopeless medically. By implication, the appeals court rejected the claim that Fox would have had the right to reject therapy in any circumstances in which his life was at stake.[75] Barring this conclusion, the court must find that Fox ought not to live anymore, whether or not he was dying. Unfortunately the court was not willing to confront this issue squarely. By refusing to do so, it gave no guidance as to the nature of the worthless life or the degree of disability that is necessary to absolve the state of its duty to preserve life.

Fundamentally, both the trial and appeals courts recognized that clear statements from the individual indicating the kind of care one wants will be present in only a very few cases. It was present in the instant case and for the court it was determinative. Nonetheless, the court's recognition that this was a special case is certainly correct. As such, the court concluded that it must offer some guidance for the more numerous cases in which such knowledge is absent.

On the crucial question at stake, however, the guidance offered by the court is plainly untenable. In attempting to delineate just when the state's role as protector of life may give way to the right of the patient to die, the court set forth this standard:

> The necessary medical criteria for the activation of the patient's right are apparent: He must be terminally ill; he must be in a vegetative coma characterized by the physician as permanent, "chronic" or "irreversible"; he must lack cognitive brain function; and the probability of his ever regaining cognitive brain function must be extremely remote. The State's interest in protecting the sanctity of life will tolerate no less stringent medical standard than this.[76]

In practical terms this is hardly intelligible. Does the court mean that the patient must be comatose, terminally ill or brain dead? These are not the same standard at all. Presumably the court did not intend *cognitive brain function* to refer to brain death standards; to what, then does that phrase refer? The court offered no guidance at this point, retreating like the journal literature into vague generalities about human functioning and the meaning of life questions on which the court has no expertise whatever.

The truth is that this is not a standard at all. It is three standards, only one of which would come close to meeting the court's own goal of "strict medical criteria." The cognitive-function standard is so loose as to offer no relevant guidance at all. Adding the notion of a comatose patient may seem to give more precise guidance at this point but only at the price of a coherent viewpoint. If the court is, as it says, concerned that the incompetent have the same rights as the competent then this addition will not do. The class of incompetent persons is far larger than the class of permanently comatose persons. One will have to give. Either we inconsistently limit the threshold or we conclude that profoundly retarded and chronically insane persons should have life-giving care withheld when they get sick.

The alternative would be to limit ourselves to terminal patients, as the trial court here wished to do. This would offer a reasonably precise medical threshold, and thus avoid the problems just noted. The court, however, was precluded from making this maneuver by its desire to help Brother Fox. At this point the appeals court bluntly states the awesome truth that others have only implied.

> The principal state interest to be protected in this proceeding . . . is the preservation of the sanctity of life. . . . Yet the patient in a permanent vegetative coma has no hope of recovery and merely lies, trapped in a technological limbo, awaiting the inevitable. As a matter of established fact such a patient has no health and in the true sense no life for the state to protect. Thus the use of a respirator or any other extraordinary means of life support, under these circumstances does not serve to advance the state's interest in protecting health or life.[77]

As disturbing as it is, this is the only way to salvage the result in *Eichner*. In fact, this is the assumption hidden in all of these cases. Though the appeal court tries to resolve the case in terms of a constitutional right to privacy, it must know that such a path is either nonsensical or unhelpful. To the extent that such a maneuver is an attempt to avoid the court's own "best interest" choice, it is plain nonsense, as we have observed above. But unless the court believes that it can avoid such a choice, the attempt to stretch the concept of privacy to cover these cases does nothing to solve the most crucial question, namely, when is it that life becomes so worthless that the state has no duty to protect it?

In upholding the judgment of the trial and appeals courts,

the state supreme court explicitly and wisely refrained from disposing of the case in terms of a constitutional right of privacy. Nevertheless, by still framing the question in terms of Brother Fox's autonomous right of choice, it actually solves none of the problems to which such a fiction gives rise in the much more numerous cases where the patient has not made an explicit choice as Brother Fox had done. Moreover, though it rejected the appeals court's elaborate process for making these decisions on behalf of another, it offered none of its own. As a result it seems unclear whether this court wished to include in its judgment the much larger group of cases in which a patient had not made known his wishes. If it did, then it must produce the very kind of substantive and procedural criteria that the appeals court unsuccessfully tried to produce.[78]

The problems in the decisions of these courts flow largely from their unwillingness to confront and resolve the most fundamental issues at stake. It is understandable that courts do not want to assume the burden of deciding when death is in someone's best interest. No one seems to know the answer to that question, especially in terms adequate to establish the precedent and policy typically expected of court decisions.

But that failure to establish precedent and policy may be the most crucial point of all. If it is impossible to answer the questions that must be answered in shaping public policies, their oblique maneuvers to fashion such policies are readily understandable. This does not however justify their attempts to resolve these issues. The confusions and contradictions in themselves are enormously problematic; as policy, they point us in directions that few really want to go. When we are told flatly by an appeals court in our second most populous state that a comatose patient has no life for the state to protect, we may begin to envision the open departure from our traditions that these courts seem about to endorse.

Herbert and *Conroy*

As this is being written, the cutting edge of the discussion both in the ethical and professional literature and in the courts concerns the possibility of removing even IV fluids and feeding tubes from incompetent patients. For such patients, are tube feeding and IV fluids always morally required, only required sometimes, or never morally required? Two court cases and a statement just released by the judicial council of the American Medical Association have served to focus the current interest in this question but these cases are by no means unique.[79] In Los Angeles two physicians were charged with murder for taking Clarence Herbert, a comatose, severely brain damaged patient off a respirator and removing his feeding tube. When taken off respiratory assistance, he unexpectedly continued to breathe on his own, hence the decision made the next day to discontinue nutritional support as well. This decision was certain to cause his death. When it did, prosecutors brought felony charges apparently on the assumption that this act was significantly different from the removal of the respirator or other mechanical assistance such as dialysis, both of which were routinely removed from incompetent, severely ill patients in California.[80]

Given Mr. Herbert's already grim medical prognosis—his coma was the result of a massive heart attack after surgery—as well as his status as a permanently comatose patient, his case did not appear to create serious moral difficulties; nor was it as immediately relevant over a wide range of analogous situations as was the case of Claire Conroy in New Jersey. Claire was an eighty-four-year-old severely demented nursing-home patient who had a typical assortment of physical diseases of old age, in her case arteriosclerotic heart disease, diabetes, and hypertension. She could move her limbs in a limited way and in response to some stimuli she would smile, moan or cry out. But though she had many ailments she could not, in any reasonable use of language be said to be terminally ill. She was simply demented and incurably ill from the typical diseases of old age. As such, her case mirrors those of hundreds of thousands of persons from the aged to the severely mentally ill.[81]

Unlike the patients in previous seminal right-to-die cases, Claire Conroy did not require the elaborate interventions of medical technology to keep her alive. She did not require the use of a respirator or dialysis or even transfusions. What she needed was food and water, the simple necessities of bodily survival: at once the most basic physical needs of each person and the easiest to provide. Unable to take food by mouth Claire had to be fed with a tube, whose removal would surely lead to her death. It was that tube which the family wanted removed. When the nursing home refused, the family went to court to compel it.

The discussion around cases like that of Claire Conroy has tended to divide between those who see her situation as qualitatively indistinguishable from that of Karen Quinlan and those who believe that food and water are the most basic sorts of human care, to be provided even when all else would be unreasonable.[82] Those in the former category may be willing to concede that we should be more reluctant to remove a feeding tube than a dialyzer but they nevertheless regard the tube as qualitatively similar. And a decision to remove the tube may be made in the light of analysis of the gravity of the patient's illness, the prospects for recovery, and the prospective quality of life of the patient.

The critics have generally argued that food and water are a basic form of care, whose provision whether to the poor, the weak, or the sick is rooted in a fundamental human moral sensitivity. It is a sensitivity that we can ill afford to treat lightly. Moreover, the argument runs, a feeding tube is not an intrusive technology that keeps going a bodily process that would otherwise stop. It is simply a means of getting food into the digestive system, a system that is itself fully functional. It is a simple matter of being unable to swallow. As such food and fluids should not be taken away from patients like Claire Conroy, even if in some such cases we should do nothing more aggressive to keep them alive, such as use a respirator.[83] These claims made by the critics are serious but they cannot ultimately be determinative. The moral sensitivity to which they rightly point is surely not just a concern for food. Care for those who are poor, or sick or handicapped is a much broader notion and a more adequate description by far of the sensitivity involved. But once we admit this broader definition of care into the argument, it may just as well be a lack of care to stop dialysis or

164

insulin or a respirator. The privileged position of food and fluids seems tenuous at best.

Moreover, it is not at all clear that tube feeding can be distinguished from other forms of treatment in the manner that the critics desire. If tube feeding must be provided, surely an oxygen mask must be used in a patient with severe emphysema or other pulmonary disease. They do the same thing: make available to the body that which it cannot obtain on its own. But what then is the meaningful difference between an oxygen mask and a respirator that simply enables the lungs to fill up with air when they lack the power to do so on their own? Finding a serious, coherent, distinction at this point is, I submit, an exercise in splitting hairs. Moreover, it is bound to seem insignificant and disingenuous, seeing the trees and deliberately missing the forest. The critics may be right, it is wrong to remove the feeding tube from Claire Conroy. But to reach that conclusion by focussing narrowly on the tube itself is hardly adequate.

The Supreme Court of New Jersey obliquely recognized this point when it considered the case. They found it impossible to distinguish in some qualitative manner between Claire Conroy and Karen Quinlan. Both patients required the assistance of technological medicine to keep them alive and in both cases the question was whether and in what fashion that technology might be withdrawn.[84]

In some respects this court is as confused as it was a decade ago in *Quinlan*. In particular it remains enamored of the transparently inadequate maneuver of trying to resolve these cases with recourse to the acknowledged right of competent patients to refuse medical care. This is nonsense and the court knows it, especially here. Competent patients can refuse any care at all, no matter how unreasonable their refusal might be. But the very point of the court setting the rigorous conditions for withholding care in the case of incompetents that it does here is to deny that any such right is at all relevant in the resolution of these cases.

The court recognizes this point in practice by providing restrictions on the withholding of treatment that are much more restrictive than those that this same court provided in *Quinlan*. Here the court sets forth a sensitive discrimination between three sorts of cases in which different standards for decision making apply:

1. subjective,
2. limited objective, and
3. pure objective.

The first case is one in which there is clear, incontrovertible evidence about the subjective choice that this patient would want made in these circumstances. Such evidence could be as a living will or another written document—a passage from a letter or the like. In the case of Brother Fox, for example, such a subjective standard was met and it was determinative.[85]

The "limited objective" standard applies to cases in which some evidence exists concerning a patient's subjective desires, but not enough to be compelling and definitive. In these cases the available subjective evidence must be complemented with a showing that the burdens of a continued life clearly outweigh the benefits to that person. When they do, and when, in addition, evidence exists that the person would have agreed, then we may presume that we are acting in accord with his choice, one that we must respect.[86]

The toughest cases are those like Claire Conroy's, where no such evidence exists at all. Here, according to the court, we are permitted to substitute our subjective judgment about "best interest" for the missing judgment of the patient. What we need, however, is a "purely objective" standard, uncontaminated by the subjective preference of the family or the physician. For the court this must involve a twofold determination. First is the benefit and burden calculation just noted. Secondly, a determination must be made that "the recurring, unavoidable and severe pain of the patient's life with treatment should be such that the effect of continuing, life sustaining treatment would be inhumane." In other words, the key to the benefit/burden test is the painfulness of the patient's continued life.[87]

If this is what the court meant to conclude, it is a major step away from *Quinlan* and post-*Quinlan* cases. It is at least plausible to presume that pain, as a sensation and as a physiological response is present when someone is in a condition that would be painful to normal adults. Thus a judgment about pain would be able to meet the court's desire for an objective standard, uncontaminated by the desires of physicians or family members. To the extent that the painfulness standard is adhered to, however, other standards that rely on preference or presumption must be set aside. Suffering, for example, is an emotional response intimately connected with the patient's desires and hopes. Without direct communication from the patient, claims about suffering are sheer presumptions so subjective in their nature as to hardly come close to the announced goal of an "objective test." So too are similar claims about "meaningless lives" or assaults on "human dignity." Both of these claims depend directly on the patients' views of themselves, their hopes, and their world: beliefs that are so personal as to be useless in the kind of determination the court wants to make, absent a clear record of these beliefs directly from the patient.

To put the matter bluntly, the test that the court sets forth in the Conroy case will not lead to the decision reached in *Quinlan*. If the feeding tube and the respirator are equivalent means of life support, as the court here believes, then the question must be resolved in terms of the *pure objective* test that the court applied to Claire Conroy. Karen Quinlan had never made her wishes known, and no credible evidence existed regarding them. Thus the key question would be the painfulness of her life; but she was not in pain. She could feel pain, which is a crucial test for distinguishing brain death from coma, but she was not in continuing pain. *Conroy* could have been derived from *Quinlan* by way of the hopelessly subjective concept of a "life not worth living," or an "unendurable" existence. But if the court rejects that move, as it does here, neither Karen nor Claire can have their life supports removed.[88]

The critics are correct; the feeding tube should not be removed from Claire Conroy, but not because the tube is part of that hopelessly elusive category of "ordinary means" and a respirator is not. Though it may not know it, this court is on the right track. Without compelling evidence of her own choice or

167

continuous, uncontrollable pain, removing the tube amounts to a purely subjective assessment of the quality of her life. This is the judgment that ought to be of most concern to the critics. But once properly thought out along the lines of *Conroy*, it is a line of inquiry fatal to most of the current discussion.

Conclusion

If the fundamental issue regarding a life not worth living cannot be answered in a manner consistent with the premises of a liberal regime and in terms precise enough to distinguish only those cases one wishes to consider reasonable deaths, then the required changes in law and public policy cannot be sustained. I submit this is true, irrespective of how strong sentiment is in any particular case. Law and policy cannot, ultimately, be wedded to the particulars of a case but must formulate general precepts to cover the great mass of men and cases. To establish a rule which leads to just results in the special case but unjust results in the typical case is to affront both law and justice.

Such seems to be the fundamental problem of reliance on courts as social policy makers. For courts are ultimately confronted with individual cases where sentiment abounds and special considerations or unusually peculiar behavior are most easily alleged. It is easy to sympathize with the plight of Karen Quinlan's parents or to grieve over her situation. What is infinitely more difficult is to generalize from her plight a policy that reaches not only her special circumstances but leads to justice for the community as well. Courts, however, are not skilled in any of the kinds of inquiry that might be required to answer the questions that necessarily arise in any attempt to put into practice any policy of euthanasia in any of its forms.

Once the fictions associated with the notion of substituted judgment are properly set aside, we can see that only one sort of right-to-die case raises fundamental issues regarding individual liberty and its relation to the doctrine of equal worth.

168

These are the cases in which a patient plainly and coherently states that he or she wants no more medical care for the disease. Of this subgroup, a still smaller number will present themselves in a fashion that may require some public resolution of competing claims. Unless the patient requires the assistance of others to remove oneself from therapy, no public issue is present and no policy needs to be established. Where the patient can do as one pleases without involving others, his or her liberty remains intact. One can do as one pleases without involving others or forcing them to make choices regarding their participation in the act.

The most difficult cases are those in which the patient clearly and coherently expresses a choice which he or she cannot carry out. At this point, someone else must ratify the decision and assist the patient in carrying it out. It is doubtful, however, whether law and public policy can here play a useful role. To provide any guidance, such a policy must either state publicly that whatever choice any patient makes for any reason will be honored, or it must distinguish the cases where a patient's decision to forego further life-sustaining care will and will not be honored. As we have already seen, the former seems patently unreasonable. Any sound public resolution of these cases requires setting forth a quality of life threshold that is both impossible to specify and inconsistent with the premises of the regime. Law and public policy are ill-advised to extend themselves into matters such as these that are beyond their competence. To specify the required criteria at law would strike at the founding principles of the regime and would almost certainly produce criteria so elastic in application as to insure serious injustice. On the other hand, some cases will arise, however few, where individual liberty is clearly at stake in an uncompromised manner, where a patient clearly, coherently, and reasonably says that he or she wants no more treatment. It is too much to ask law and policy to override liberty in these cases, however much the case may, in theory, resemble suicide. While law cannot sanction such choices explicitly without moving into the turbulent waters of the life not worth living, neither should law require or be enforced in such a manner as to produce the deprivations of liberty that would occur if treatment were forced on someone in such a case.

The strictness of the principles of common law applied logically to these cases stems from the belief in the worth of each life—a belief that lies at the core of western democratic civilization. The stringency of such principles sustains that reverence for life and makes it a force in public choices and private decision making. While in some cases of the type we considered here, strict enforcement of the terms within which this reverence is couched may strike too deeply at individual liberty, the terms themselves are not therefore impotent. Even when we ultimately decide in favor of individual liberty, the presence of law itself forces us to take more seriously then we might the awesome decisions faced by the patient and the physician. When a patient cries out that he or she wants no more life-saving or sustaining medical care, the physician must not give in to that request without the most profound meditation on that decision, sustained by a reverence for all human life that is established in public law and professional codes.

When the liberty of the patient is not at stake, law and policy must speak for life, untempered by the profound concern for individual liberty that our regime fosters. Since the various maneuvers by which choice is attributed to the incompetent patient typically are sheer fictions, they must be dismissed as evasive. Once they are set aside, however, the choice to withdraw clearly life-preserving therapy from an incompetent patient is reduced to the stark quality of life decision for which no one has been able to provide compelling criteria in either legal or moral terms. Without such criteria, abuses of discretion and unfairness will abound: this point was seen in the discussion of infanticide as well. It is little wonder, therefore, that law and policy have not until recently and should not now attempt to sanction such choices.

Of course many of these decisions will need to be made with imperfect medical data. Often we will simply not know whether a proposed therapy will preserve a patient's life, or whether it will shorten his or her life, or whether it will merely

prolong an already inevitable process of dying. These uncertainties are treated at greater length in the final chapter. Law
and policy cannot take account of such nuances in individual
cases. Such are matters for the clinician and the like. The most
that can be done in law and policy—and even in general moral
theory—is to articulate the direction in which deliberation
should proceed and to show that some alternatives are unacceptable at the outset. In other words, we can point the direction in which a proper answer to these cases of uncertainty will
be found, but without the specific nuances of the case at hand
we can do no more. Similarly, law and policy can exclude the
unacceptable and give public articulation to our core beliefs and
deepest sentiments; but law and policy are incapable of deciding before hand in these cases of indecision and uncertainty.
We will return to these matters later.[89]

CHAPTER FIVE

Suicide

Introduction

"There is but one truly serious philosophical problem," wrote Albert Camus, "and that is suicide. Whether life is or is not worth living amounts to answering the fundamental question of philosophy."[1] As a proposition regarding the nature of philosophic inquiry, Camus's assertion is entirely on the mark. The question of suicide does strike at the heart of the human predicament. It raises the central questions of human existence in the most compelling manner possible, questions which, before recent analytic fads, were and remain central in philosophic inquiry. Suicide in particular has been richly examined by most of the greatest philosophers of the western tradition and in recent times it has proved to be an endlessly fascinating subject for certain philosophic traditions and segments of popular thought.[2] Despite this fascination with suicide in certain circles, it has not been a controversial issue in law and policy. To be sure, sociologists have, since the time of Durkheim, studied the social phenomenon and psychiatrists have explored its intrapsychic dimensions and have set forth numerous measures to reduce its sorrowful influence.[3] But the questions that ani-

173

mated Camus and his progenitors were barely mentioned by sociologists, psychiatrists and policy writers. From the point of view of public policy and professional practice, this is, I submit, a correct starting point. For whatever metaphysical mileage may be gained from meditation on the meaning and worth of human life, it is indisputably true that the founding and sustaining of a decent, humane political order already presupposes an answer to Camus's question: life is worth living.

Nonetheless, suicide is an issue that lies at the center of our concerns in this book. Of all the situations where life and death are in the balance, suicide seems to raise most directly the question of individual liberty—the right of the individual to live and die as he chooses. We hardly need be reminded that such liberty is deeply cherished in democratic societies and has special resonance in periods such as ours where even the most minimal liberties are routinely denied to hundreds of millions of people governed by powerful and despotic regimes.

Humean Natural Right to Suicide

At first glance, suicide seems not to involve the problematic situation where one person must choose death for another. Nor, need it even involve another in aiding or giving effect to a choice thus made. Suicide seems to present itself as the act of the free individual par excellence, disconnected from a wider context of faithful conviction, communal values or public concerns. Suicide appears as the pristine example of human freedom and it is in this context that many modern writers have defended the right to commit suicide against what they believe were the biases of conventional morality and religious superstition. Especially since the appearance of Hume's celebrated essay many have been convinced that suicide represents one of the most fundamental of man's natural rights.[4] To argue against such a right has appeared to be an attack on liberty in the name of religious bigotry. This theme is carried through by many philosophers such as Nietzsche and by contemporary libertarian psychiatrists such as Szaz and Slater.[5] Essentially the point is the same: suicide is the consummate expression of the liberty

174

that is characteristic of the natural state of man. This primordial right of man must be respected by the social and political order within which the individual lives. As such, policy and practice permitting civil intervention with potential suicides is little more than a revised version of the religious tyrannies of the past.[6]

Szaz's Restatement

In his trenchant essay on the subject Szaz himself has offered us a classic statement of this right:

> A man's life belongs to himself. Hence, he has the right to take his own life, that is commit suicide. To be sure, this view recognizes that a man may have a moral responsibility to his family and others and that by killing himself he reneges on these responsibilities. But these are moral wrongs that society in its corporate capacity as the state cannot properly punish. Hence the state must eschew attempts to regulate such behavior by means of formal sanction such as criminal or mental hygiene laws.[7]

Just as in Hume suicide is here seen fundamentally as a matter of private natural right. To control suicide is to control this liberty, a matter of the gravest moral consequence. "I would maintain," writes Slater, "that the right to die transcends the claims of family and society. A man's life is his own and if we say it is not we are saying he is a slave and not a free man."[8] As a matter of private right, no one ought to have one's suicidal acts interfered with so long as the individual is the only target of one's violence.

Though pressed with vigor of late this argument is deeply flawed in several ways. From Hume onward the most fundamental error has been to confuse the natural man with the citizen and thence to deduce sound public policy from man's supposed natural rights. Out of this mixture comes the claim that whatever rights man had in the state of nature, they must form the assumptions from which public policy on any of these matters is developed. In the instant case, if man had a natural right to kill himself, then he must have that same right as a citizen.

175

Modern philosophers, of course, have conceived of man as an independent self, a transcendental ego whose nature is displayed precisely in one's freedom from natural virtue or human convention. As the master of its own fate the liberated self knows no constraints except those imposed by the self constructed law of the willing subject. Furthermore, by understanding that the individual exists prior to and independently of the family, the city and the divine modernity comes to view morality as fundamentally protecting the privacy of many to preserve the privacy of the self. Rules come to be viewed as the essence of morality and to be formulated precisely to protect the aloneness of the individual. Obedience to rules becomes the standard of virtue and virtue is redefined as the disposition to obey.[9]

The inescapable privatization of the suicidal act that follows from these premises finds its apogee in a recent article where it is maintained that we must simply accept the subjective, even incoherent rationales of suicidal persons. Supposedly we all experience reality differently. One man's minor discomfort is another man's major distress. When my reality is sufficiently distressful to me, suicide is, *eo ipso*, permissible without the addition of any further reasons. Here the appeal to privacy is no longer merely a claim to be let alone; it has ended in an appeal to a solipsistic world of private meaning interpretable only by the individual, a world where any reason or none is sufficient. What is reasonable or justified is made dependent on the whims of the psychotic and the depressed. He cannot even speak of reason or rationality for to do so presumes the very shared reality that this author denies.[10]

In this result the privatization of morality and the epistemic skepticism first announced by the founders of modern thought reach their ultimate conclusion about suicide. We can no longer even speak to the suicidal individual on this account. The supposedly solitary act of suicide is given meaning only by the private language of the suicidal man. The privatization of the act itself is mirrored in the privatization of the meaning by which we understand it. Lacking a shared meaning silence prevails, broken only by the contradictory speech of those, who presumably seek to announce the end of speech concerning suicide.

But granting all of this does not necessarily entail any conclusions regarding the question of how we shall deal with suicide as a matter of public policy. Natural rights do not necessarily make civic rights. In fact the very point of contract theory is the disparity between nature and convention in this regard. The exercise of all of man's natural powers to their fullest is incompatible with the requirements of communal life and such an exercise must be tempered in the transition from nature to community.[11] To confuse the natural and the civil state is to ignore this difference, a distinction on which stands the possibility of a humane society.

At this point the maneuver from nature to convention as in the tradition from Hume is beset with two areas of confusion. First, it must be assumed that actual persons are sufficiently like the semi-artificial constructs that inhabit the state of nature in modern political philosophy for there to be any reason to believe that they can exercise the same rights. Certainly pre-Rawlsian contract theorists populated the state of nature with human beings whose passions, interests, and fears mirrored those found in most actual human beings. In this regard the maneuver from nature to convention seems plausible. One searches in vain, however, for one of these savage people who is incapable of calculating the best pursuit of individual interests, given passion and fear. None of these hypothetical Adams or Eves appears retarded, demented or even depressed. They are burdened with none of the mental or physical disorders that commonly distort our view of life and lead some individuals to conclude that theirs is worthless.

To transfer the right to kill oneself from nature to society requires transferring this natural man as well. This is, of course, the deeper meaning of the widely accepted notion that the individual must be competent to choose suicide in a manner that we ought to respect and allow. In other words, he must be a rational calculator—that is, one who is not coerced into such a choice.[12] This conclusion is obliquely admitted even by Szaz and his followers who either deny the reality of mental illness itself or else deny that there is any correlation between mental illness and suicide. Thus most of those who do kill themselves will supposedly be the fully rational calculator of liberal theory. As one set of Szazian authors recently wrote: "Most people who commit suicide are not mentally ill."[13] The importance of this claim to the Szazian position seems obvious. No one wants a person to kill himself for frivolous or erroneous reasons, especially not when one's capacity to know the weakness of one's reasons for killing himself is compromised. At this point the Szazian defender has two options. He may give up one's claim about the natural right to commit suicide forming the basis of policy or he can hold to the sorts of assumptions regarding mental illness to which we just called attention.

Reality of Mental Illness

Unfortunately, this claim regarding the mental state of suicidal persons is plainly false. A relationship between suicide and mental illness has been found everywhere the matter has been studied. Consider, for example, just the important study of Barraclough and his associates in England. In this retrospective analysis of 100 cases of completed suicide only one case was found where no symptoms of mental illness could be documented. On the basis of the interviews with family and friends well over 80 per cent of the victims of suicide could be reasonably diagnosed as suffering from a specific mental disease.[14] The other studies from Europe and the United States showing a similar relationship need not be reviewed here.[15] Suffice it to say that this assertion is false.

Once these facts become clear the weakness of the Szazian position becomes apparent. In the sorts of cases that are by far the most common the person is not the calculator of liberal theory. In practice, Szaz's view leads not to man's freedom from religious prejudice but to one's bondage to the passions and ills of mortality. But this bondage limits human autonomy as much or more than any despot. It is a tyranny of its own, distorting the mind and limiting the will in ways that are subtle, profound and often pervasive. When this picture of actual suicidal persons becomes clear, the difference between these cases and other sorts of issues involving individual liberty becomes readily apparent. For example, one often-heard argument regarding the immorality of coercive suicide intervention was recently stated this way:

> Is involuntary civil commitment of the mentally ill on the grounds of dangerousness to self morally justifiable? The question posed by Livermore Malmquist and Meehl surely answers itself: "if in the criminal law it is better that ten guilty men go free than that one innocent man suffer, how can we say in civil commitment that it is better that fifty-four harmless people be incarcerated lest one dangerous man be free?[16]

Such an analogy to the criminal justice system is very tenuous at best. Suicidal persons are not accused persons whose liberty is being restricted as a means of punishment. In whatever language they are described they remain sick, disturbed human beings, irrespective of whether they do try to kill themselves again. Allowing these people to remain sick and disturbed would do little to foster their ability to make truly autonomous choices free from the limitations of their illness. This is especially true for victims of mental disease with its attendant distortions of perception, cognition and will.[17] As such I think it can be reasonably maintained that even if the value of autonomy were as great as the above argument implies, it is not harmed by proper psychiatric hospitalization in anything approaching the degree implied above.

One might attempt to salvage this transition from natural man to civil man with the claim that the maneuver is only an assumption made necessary by the injustices that would follow if we assumed that suicidal persons are mentally ill. In this case the claim would be that we have no reliable means of predicting who will and who will not commit suicide and of helping those who might. As a result many people will have their liberty coercively interfered with as a means of preventing suicides by using unproven or ineffective therapies.[18] If this is the case it would seem most reasonable to make the assumption concerning the suicidal person which we have just criticized, even if in some few cases it is inaccurate.

Unfortunately, this sort of shift does not salvage the position. It may be that the ability of professionals to predict that a specific person will kill himself is unacceptably low.[19] This, however, is the wrong question. If our concern is with the unjust interference with human liberty the proper question must be the ability of professionals to diagnose mental disease and offer effective treatment that will restore as much functional autonomy as possible to the individual! Therefore, in my view, the morality of intervention is intimately connected to the seriously diminished capacity for autonomous choice and action in the vast majority of those who commit or attempt suicide and the correlative ability of professionals to treat mental illness and restore a measure of autonomous functioning to the patient.

Unlike suicide prediction, however, the data demonstrating substantial ability on the part of professionals in this regard is clear and uncontestable. If accepted, it suggests that the proper description of policies that permit the hospitalization of suicidal persons is to say that we are hospitalizing a number of sick human beings, many of whom will be treated with some success and some of whom will be helped to avoid the suicide that would otherwise be the final outcome of their illness. To reject this description is to reject the category of mental illness, a point not at issue here. The consistent finding of a link between suicide and mental illness or the evidence regarding the abilities of professionals to diagnose and treat this sort of disease, makes it evident that none of these moves is likely to be tenable.[20]

Religious Critique of Natural Right to Suicide

The second confusion between the natural and the conventional state that is inherent in this position is more serious and theoretically dubious. This concerns the notion of natural rights and their role in the formation of policy. In the tradition from Hume it was supposed that natural rights are moral claims of individuals that are prior to and independent of social and communal life. Hence, supposedly, they must be the basis of acceptable public law. The problematic status of such a maneuver, however, was recognized even by the founders of liberal contract theory, in two fundamental ways. In the first place, none of the great theorists of the contract tradition ever conceived of the actual existence of prepolitical men and women supposedly endowed with substantial moral claims, waiting to join a society that would protect their rights. In this respect they all conceived of natural rights in a fashion specifically designed to support and sustain the existence of liberal, limited government. Like the notion of equality, the claim of natural rights is something of a construct, a necessary premise of what is to follow, but which is not properly viewed as the immediate basis of individual moral claims or obligations or of public policies and laws. Locke again is precisely on target, though his views are reflected in many others, such as Hobbes, Grotius, Blackstone and Kant. In the celebrated opening chapters of the Second Treatise, Locke posits equality as the basis of liberal democratic regimes. As we saw earlier this is the premise on which he bases a commitment to individual liberty and the free societies that protect it. From this premise Locke then draws out two sorts of natural rights. The first are those rights that inhere in the individual equally as an expression of his moral or civil standing. Secondly, the individual has rights of self-defense and punishment as means of protecting himself from others who would deprive him of the core rights that define his equal standing with others, such as by enslaving or murdering him.[21]

In the transition from the state of nature to civil society, the individual justifiably relinquishes his right of punishment and much of his right of self-defense in exchange for a respite from the perpetual state of war that exists when these rights are continually exercised in the state of nature by each individual. In this context, however, Locke maintains that the core rights are inalienable, since they provide the ground for the most basic limitations on government.[22] Since the core rights are inalienable, there are two things which, according to Locke, a person may never justifiably do: sell himself into slavery or commit suicide. This conclusion seems to follow since both slavery and suicide are the fundamental ways in which one can

181

irreparably alienate either one's liberty or one's right to life. It is not at all obvious, however, that Locke's position regarding the status of suicide as a natural right is as straightforward as it seems here.

On the surface Locke connects his teaching concerning suicide with a religious doctrine regarding man's status as a creature of God. Man is said to be God's "workmanship," "made to last during His, not another's, pleasure."[23] This view of man as the property of the divine, of course, requires theistic premises to make it work. But on a close examination no adequate justification of such premises can be found in the whole of Locke's philosophic teaching. In the *Essay Concerning Human Understanding*, he adduces various proofs for the existence of God. But these proofs are quite inadequate for the task of justifying theism, let alone demonstrating the truth of the specific theistic beliefs one finds in the teaching on suicide.[24] In his discussion of Christian doctrine proper, no proof of theism is even attempted and the theology itself contains no such doctrine of man as the property of God.[25] In fact the best view of Locke's whole theistic teaching is to regard it as an important political myth, necessary as myth but incapable of being demonstrated in scientific terms.

Secular Meaning of Traditional Teaching

If this is the proper context in which to understand Locke's teaching on suicide, the core of that teaching becomes clear: it is a political teaching intimately connected to the concerns of the book from whence it comes. Locke teaches that, whatever may be true of human capacities in a hypothetical state of nature, the assertion that a man's life is worthless is incompatible with the premise of equal worth on which liberal societies are founded. It is a teaching that leads us to consider what public policy regarding suicide must be, not necessarily what rights the human being may have had in the state of nature. The belief in the equal worth of each human life renders the testimony of the suicidal man both suspect and dangerous as the basis of public policy. To adopt his view of the matter essentially denies his equal worth. To accept what he proposes to do with his belief in life's worthlessness is to accept the alienation of his most fundamental right, simply because he asserts that it will be better this way. The essence of the liberal conviction regarding inalienable rights has, as we saw in a previous chapter, dissolved at this point.[26]

Locke's teaching on suicide is thus directly connected to the concerns of civil society and the public values which must support it. Whether, on some grounds, suicide is intrinsically immoral or is always morally prohibited is a question that Locke simply does not treat. But he does sever the necessity of any connection between an answer to this question and the question of how public law and policy should treat suicide. For Locke, to suggest that the regime should set forth in public law the belief that the individual could alienate one's most fundamental right whenever one wanted was to teach a doctrine that presupposes the incorrectness of the premises of liberal regimes. The implications of such questions about the public life of liberal regimes is a matter we have examined in an earlier chapter but we can now see the importance of that analysis in considering what kinds of policy questions are raised by suicide and suicide intervention programs.

In severing this connection between pure natural right and acceptable public policy the greatest modern philosophers point to the fundamental weaknesses of the positions taken by Hume and Szaz. Policies must be shaped with a watchful eye on the situations where they will be employed and the people who will employ them. Concerning suicide we are thus pointed toward the broader context of a teaching concerning the worthlessness of some lives—a necessary part of Szaz's view—and to the actual state of those who come to feel thus about themselves. On both grounds it seems that the pure "natural right" championed by the libertarian tradition from Hume to Szaz fails as an adequate policy.

Liberal and Classical Views of Suicide

By placing his teaching concerning suicide in the context of religious myth, however, Locke also points to a deeper truth than may be supposed on a single reading of the text or a superficial understanding of the mythic character of Locke's religious teaching. The religious doctrine to which he refers conceives of man as God's creature, his "product," so to speak. This general view is open to several different interpretations. Locke himself specifically connects it to man's being appointed or called to a certain station in mortality that he may not abandon without permission. To abandon one's post in the face of hardship would, in this view, amount to a failure of the courage which seems essential in the virtuous life and, more importantly, is a necessary attribute of democratic citizenship.[27] In this regard, Locke's myth mirrors the understanding of suicide that one finds in the ancients and is illuminated by Socrates' refusal to sanction it under any circumstances.[28] Like Locke's, Socrates' teaching is shrouded in religious myth concerning man's divine appointment. As in Plato's other myths, however, the religious surface both reveals and conceals a more fundamental teaching about man and his civic and cosmic condition.

This teaching, like the Stoic, was centrally directed at the outset to the problem of public virtue, the virtue of the many which alone made decent human life possible. Death itself should not be feared but suicide was different. The suicidal person admits that life is worthless, that nothing more can be done to render it bearable. This admission denies both the order of the cosmos and the order of the city in deference to the disorder of the individual self.

Like the refusal to heed Crito's advice, the prohibition of suicide announced by Socrates bears witness to the order of the city and the cosmos. Whether it be true that "everything in the universe is arranged in accordance with the good" may be debated endlessly by philosophers.[29] But Socrates is surely correct in teaching that decent life in community depends on a shared conviction that something of this sort is the case. The suicidal man testifies to a rejection of this belief. He supposedly knows that for him existence is not organized for the good or even the tolerable. Once we acknowledge the reasonableness of this assertion, we engage ourselves in his belief. As Plato well knew, such an engagement on the part of the city would do little to encourage the feeble commitment of ordinary people to justice and virtue, even virtues limited to the abilities of the many. Though they are distinct, the order of the city is coeval with the order of the cosmos. The city exists to foster human life and fulfillment. This possibility depends on the assumption by the many that the order of the cosmos is a fact. Without the belief that life is generally good they would find nothing worthwhile to nourish in the city and its very *raison d'être* would cease. But for the suicidal man life has become worthless and the mythic opinion supporting the life of the city and its members is what Hume derisively called it—superstition. For the city to remain idle or tolerant at this point is to affirm the legitimacy of the vision of man and cosmos inherent in suicide. That is why the city, even the imperfect city, cannot permit proper burial of the suicide. To do so memorializes for the many this vision of the world, a vision that denies the possibility of a humane city which alone nourishes the lives of the many themselves.[30] Plato does not teach that every conceivable act of suicide is wrong. Rather, he teaches that what matters is the opinion of the many on the broad outlines of the question. Therefore, the discussion in the *Phaedo* remains in the context of a religious myth from which he only departs in the most oblique manner. Once we have settled the question of opinion, which by its nature deals only with general cases, we will have time enough to deal privately with special cases and problems.

The order of the cosmos and the city are surely important, but the deepest truth about suicide is that it testifies to the disorder of the soul. This teaching, paradoxically, lies so near the surface of the *Apology* and the Platonic dialogues that we may be tempted to ignore it. Throughout the dialogues on the trial and death of Socrates the problem of fear and courage in the face of death recurs continually. In the *Apology* Socrates even employs a military analogy so similar in its import to the religious myth of the *Phaedo* as to be recognized by even the most casual reader. In both cases the fundamental alternatives are courage and cowardice. Not the courage to die but the courage to be is at stake in both instances.[31] To take life at the price of cowardice is to render meaningless the whole Socratic teaching regarding human virtue. This alternative is refused in the *Apology*. To take life as worthless, however, symbolizes the cowardice of those who cannot bear difficulties and misfortunes. Nowhere does Socrates speak of the courage to die in the sense of Nietzsche or Sartre; rather, his military analogy suggests the true emphasis on the courage to remain at one's post that is the basis of the teaching throughout. It is this courage that is the basis of both the order of the soul and the health of the city. On such a courageous pursuit of excellence rests the possibility of attaining true virtue and wisdom. But the military analogy also shows the connection between individual courage and the city, without which life is impossible. Unless the many believe that their lives are generally worthwhile, they will be ill-disposed to defend themselves against oppression and tyranny. In this way the Socratic emphasis on courage and the religious myth in which it is cloaked point to the intimate interconnections of self, society, and cosmos and the fundamental break with this order represented by the suicidal person.

The "New Consensus"

If the pure Szazian position goes too far, perhaps we need only modify it slightly. Such a maneuver might account for the most obvious difficulties we have seen without abandoning the essential premises regarding the natural rights of the individual. Several authors have recently developed such modified views; we may designate them as forming a "new consensus" on the question of suicide as a matter of public concern. The essential step in this revision is the claim that the right to commit suicide should be regarded as a *prima facie* right that might be overridden by any of several other moral considerations.[32]

In a recent discussion Karen Lebacqz and Tristram Englehardt state this position in lucid terms:

> We will make a modest argument in favor of the right of persons to dispose of their own lives . . . to take this approach is to suggest that suicide should be reasonable un-

less sufficient reason can be found why it is not. It is, therefore, to put the burden of proof on those who oppose suicide rather than on those who defend it. As Flew suggests, "It is up to any person and any institution wanting to prevent anyone from doing anything he wishes to do to provide positive good reason to justify that interference." The fundamental principle of liberty is taken as constitutive of human life and meaning. Since arguments in principle against suicide do not succeed, there is a *prima facie* right to kill oneself.[33]

The essential premises of Hume's position remain intact. The individual is still conceived of as having a natural right to kill himself whenever he finds life burdensome. But most of the "new consensus" writers wish to avoid the excesses of the Szazian position both in moral and policy terms. In moral terms Lebacqz and Englehardt argue that while a man or woman has this natural right, any of several other considerations typically intervene to make it morally unjustified to commit suicide in a specific instance. In other words, in general, human beings ought not to kill themselves. After sorting out the various claims that might affect a choice for suicide, they conclude that there are three cases in which suicide which may be morally right: voluntary euthanasia, covenantal suicide, and symbolic protest.[34] The third case is easily recognized, even if obscurely defended. One kills oneself to make a larger point about social injustice. The first and second cases revolve around an understanding of one's moral or "covenantal obligations." In the first case the individual is incapable of fulfilling any obligations to others and so has no countervailing claims that might override the natural right to kill oneself. In the second case the individual kills oneself as a means of fulfilling some covenantal obligation: for example, the case of "the self-sacrificial suicide of one who chooses to die rather than to burden her family or friends." To turn any of these categories into a policy of nonintervention or assistance in either law or morality, as these authors wish to do, will require a clear, coherent delineation of each sort of case so that we will know when intervention is justified or where legal sanctions against those who assist in suicide are appropriate. But none of these cases is defined with a close approximation of the precision requisite for public policy.

Consider, for example, the case of "voluntary euthanasia." They write about it as follows:

> Under certain circumstances, such as terminal illness accompanied by great pain, it may be impossible to fulfill normal covenantal obligations to one's family and friends. If so, these obligations cease and thus the right to dispose of one's own life is not contravened by any restraining duties. In these circumstances the right to suicide cannot be defeated because the circumstances themselves defeat the possibility of fulfilling any obligations to others.[35]

The vagueness in this passage renders it very unsound as a guide for action. We have no idea which obligations are those whose fulfillment must be impossible for suicide to be morally permitted. Is one enough? Suppose a man is bedridden yet has the capacity to smile and talk occasionally. Is suicide justified because he can no longer fulfill many of his obligations to support and provide for his family? One interpretation of the passage would be that the last sentence commits them to hold that the capacity to fulfill any obligation is sufficient. On this interpretation, however, the cogency of the position vanishes. For there simply will be no individuals who both can deliberate and choose and yet cannot fulfill any obligations to others.

Furthermore, the logic of this position appears shaky. The mere fact that a person does not fulfill one's obligations will not do. One must be incapable of doing so. Since these authors sanction suicide and assisting in suicide, this judgment of incapacity would have to be a communal judgment But once we have decided when death is acceptable over life and when we may aid someone to kill oneself, such a judgment certainly applies to many human beings. At this point these authors provide no reason beyond mere assertion for not endorsing nonvoluntary euthanasia of all those who meet the given criteria but who cannot offer consent, such as severely retarded persons, and who cannot do the deed themselves. In short, the logic of the position seems to represent a wholesale departure from some of our most deeply held convictions concerning the rights of and care due to severely retarded and disabled persons as well as to others who might fit into the class of being unable to fulfill their covenantal obligations.

Another version of this maneuver is to combine a list of specific cases in which suicide seems reasonable with a requirement that the person must be rational in choosing to kill himself. Otherwise intervention will be justified. A recent suggestion to develop public policy and law along these lines, however, demonstrates the severe difficulties of producing a coherent and relevant set of specific cases. The core of this suggestion is that there are specific types of cases where suicide is acceptable. They define these as cases of "irreversible and severely crippling, debilitating or painful illness or injury and cases of severe, prolonged or untreatable depression."[36] On inspection this is far too vague to be of much help. If the authors mean that the desire to die is untreatable, then a justification for such a claim will need to be offered. *Prima facie,* suicidal thoughts and behavior are treatable and it is not at all clear how we might discriminate between those that are and those that are not without the kind of intensive therapy that might be needed.

Qualifying this list of cases with the notion that the person must be rational is of no help and appears contradictory. These authors reduce the assumption about rationality to the claim that the individual ought not to suffer from "emotional stress" or "mental disease."[37] But it is unlikely that we will find any suicidal persons who are not suffering from some "emotional stress." For example, it is hard to conceive of a permanently crippled person who would not suffer emotional stress as a result. The utility of this as a discriminating criterion for public policy and professional practice is severely compromised. What we would need to know is when suicide is reasonable and that we have found to be a hopeless task insofar as we are concerned to produce criteria useful for practice. Absent such criteria any attempt to distinguish among cases of suicide where intervention is permissible and where it is not will likely be difficult if not futile.

Since such standards will not do, two alternatives appear

possible as maneuvers to salvage the "new consensus" position. First, one may give up the search for acceptable criteria for judging a suicidal act and endorse a Szazian public policy. Since moral judgment is not a matter of public policy, anyone ought to be able to kill oneself for any reason. This is the route Lebacqz and Englehardt seem to take. As a matter of public policy they would have us respect any choice for suicide and anyone's aiding someone else in giving effect to a choice he or she makes. The essential position is the solipsistic claim that "only the individual can decide what balance of freedom and life constitutes the best choices for her."[38] The individual is the only one who can determine whether his or her life is worth it. This maneuver supposedly circumvents the search for criteria by admitting that we cannot give any and asserting that we do not need to. To be successful, however, the maneuver must be maintained in all cases: the individual must always be regarded as the best judge of the worth of her own life. To assert a less comprehensive version would require the same public criteria that these authors eschew. But the stronger version seems obviously false, and is likely to be especially false about severely depressed persons contemplating suicide.

Furthermore, it is difficult to see what argument might be given for such a claim that would not also entail the view that the individual is the best judge of the moral obligations one faces and their relative strengths. Since on this account the individual is to be regarded as the best judge of one's own ranking of values, this conclusion cannot be avoided. But if true, it renders any judgment about the morality of individual suicides impossible. We could not say "you believed that this was a valid case of covenantal suicide, but you are wrong for the following reasons." But this latter statement seems to be what was intended in the claim that there are certain situations in which suicide was right and others in which it was wrong. If they wish to hold that we can make such judgments then the view that the individual is always the best judge of her ranking of values must be given up.

Most "new consensus" authors obliquely admit these points. Lebacqz and Englehardt wish to restrict the right to make such choices to persons who are "competent" to do so. "In a culture that places freedom of choice among the most important of all values," one author wrote recently, "the state has no plausible interest in preventing suicide by competent people. . . . The state should intervene to prevent suicide where the individual lacks the capacity or competence to make a choice in the matter."[39] In this way it is thought that one can provide criteria for public policy and professional practice that supposedly do not entail a moral judgment concerning the individual's decision to kill oneself.

There are two ways in which this maneuver may be made. First, one may focus on competency *per se:* the competent individual should be allowed to kill oneself if one chooses. On the other hand, one might focus on specific clinical states like intoxication that are known to produce incompetency and permit intervention only in cases where the given state exists. The first maneuver, focusing on competency *per se* will require the assumption that we can assess a person's competency to engage in an act independently of any judgment regarding the act itself. This assumption is difficult to sustain, especially about suicidal persons.[40]

Consider first the noetic component of competency. The severely depressed person may have a rather truthful picture of the immediate situation. It may be true that at that moment one has no friends or family and feels no love from any source. At a certain point one may lack the very things that make life meaningful for many people. The problem, however, is that such a person cannot envision transforming the situation by one's own effort or with the help of others. Yet, although one knows one's immediate circumstances, I seriously doubt that we are ready to give aid or comfort to such a person in committing suicide, no matter how realistic this knowledge may be. It is not a question of insanity or inebriation, but a question of reasonableness. At the point where a decision must be made, we simply cannot find a minimally sufficient level of reasonableness in the contemplated suicide to withhold our intervention.

It therefore appears that the common understanding of competency, namely that an individual knows what one is doing, is inadequate for the task assigned it. This can be seen with the help of a case that is all to familiar.

> Mr. N was a thirty-six-year-old man suffering from severe depression. He had been hospitalized five times in the past six years for the same problem. On this admission he has been markedly depressed on all major clinical indicators— anhedonia, anorexia, sleep disturbance, and so forth—and has severe feelings of helplessness and hopelessness. He is started on antidepressant drugs and group therapy. At the end of his first full week in the hospital he is sent on a weekend pass. His mother, with whom he has lived for ten years, will have nothing more to do with him so he goes to stay with his sister and brother-in-law. They have reluctantly agreed to this just for the weekend but have made it clear that they will not offer care on a long-term basis.
>
> The sister is unexpectedly called to work on Saturday and Mr. N is sent to his mother's house for the weekend. At the end to the weekend he does not want to go back to the hospital. The mother is completely fed up with him and calls the police. They come, use physical force, handcuff the man and take him back to the hospital. The next morning Mr. N feels completely abandoned by his family and feels no care or love from any source. For him life is hopeless. He asks the nurse to drive him to a bridge to jump off. When she protests he says calmly that he will write out a note stating that he asked her to do this, then she will not get into trouble.

Mr. N knew perfectly well what he was doing and why. He was correct about his family and his friends. He did lack friends and his family had rejected him in a violent manner. If we morally refuse to drive him to the bridge that can only be because we cannot accept the assertion that it would be minimally reasonable for a man in this condition to commit suicide. At that point it is just phenomenologically unsound to say that we are judging something other than the contemplated suicide itself.

Even in the rare case where one might conclude from an objective point of view that suicide might be acceptable, a closer examination will often suggest the opposite. This is seen in the following case.

Mr. A was a fifty-two-year-old white male who had been diagnosed as having Buerger's disease six years previously. This is a progressive vascular degeneration in which the patient progressively loses the use of his extremities and they must be amputated. Eventually the degenerative process reaches the brain and the patient dies. Mr. A has already had both of his legs amputated, and some loss of function was beginning to appear in the left arm. He was brought to the hospital in a severely depressed and acutely suicidal state. During the first three weeks in the hospital he remained acutely suicidal, and even attempted suicide once. After the failed attempt his mood and affect changed dramatically. He was no longer preoccupied with suicide and began to work with the local association that aided crippled persons. He was a very intelligent, extremely well-read person and his prior business expertise was a great asset to the group.

Six months later he was readmitted to the hospital in an acute suicidal state, having stopped eating six days before admission. During the hospitalization he even showed the nursing staff how he planned to kill himself by saving up his medication for an overdose. Again, however, he recovered from this episode with marked improvement in mood, affect and general functioning. This time he was discharged to an intermediate care nursing facility to live and work with other disabled persons.

He was readmitted a third time for depression and severe suicidal preoccupation. A very similar pattern of events ensued. After about a month his depressive episode lifted and his suicidal thoughts disappeared. During each suicidal episode he claimed that the one reason he had not't committed suicide yet was his orthodox Jewish faith which strictly prohibited it. He had consulted his rabbi on the matter and was counseled against suicide in religious terms.

Objectively, one might argue that if there was a case where suicide may be reasonable, this man's situation might fit. He has a progressive degenerative disease in which dementia followed by death are inevitable. His physicians have given him an estimate that he may have only three more years to live.

Even admitting all of this, however, it is clear that this individual has made no such choice for himself. His attempts to kill himself are gestures designed to call attention to his plight, not a serious and sustained choice for death. A person as intelligent and well-read as he would surely know that if he stopped eating for a week, he would be brought to the hospital, and that showing the nurses how he intended to commit suicide would only result in his cache of pills being taken away. Given this understanding of the actual context of the case, it seems clear that we should continue to treat this man and to work through future depressive episodes as has been done in the past. This man is clearly ambivalent about his desires: when and if he decides on suicide, he will not show up at the hospital or let himself be brought to the hospital for treatment; he will show up dead on arrival.

Shifting our attention from the noetic to the volitional capacities of the patient serves the new consensus position no better. It may be claimed that persons incapable of voluntary choice cannot act for themselves and are thus in a position in which we need not respect what they say or do regarding suicide and our efforts at intervention. As applied to suicide intervention this would focus attention on the capacity for choice retained by the patient, such as a patient who hears voices telling him or her to kill himself. As a general means of salvaging the competency criterion, however, this maneuver quickly leads to serious difficulties.

The case of Mr. N is useful here also. If we conclude that he is capable of choice, those who focus solely on this criterion would have us let him kill himself; many would add that we should help him kill himself. But this seems patently unreasonable, given the possibilities of treating his depressive illness. But if we conclude that his depressive disease diminishes his volitional capacities, then that claim will, in all likelihood, apply to nearly everyone who actually commits suicide. The number of persons who commit suicide and do not display signs and symptoms of serious mental illness is very small and it is reduced even further by considering those who feel coerced into suicide attempts by situational pressures.[41] Surely these

194

would be paradigm cases of persons not acting freely in a choice for suicide. But if they are removed, the number of competent suicides drops to near zero, and the utility of competency criterion in shaping public policy along "new consensus" lines seems to disappear.

At this point a second option is to focus on specific clinical states known to be associated with incompetence on any reasonable definition of these terms. Mental instability and ignorance, as one writer has recently suggested, are plainly inadequate for these purposes. As noted before almost everyone who commits suicide displays some signs or symptoms of mental instability. Such a standard would therefore sanction almost no suicides. To make it more serviceable, one would need some other criteria that would help us determine when suicide is reasonable.

The next plausible move at this point is the suggestion that intoxication with drugs or alcohol is the only condition that would warrant suicide intervention. On this account a person who is intoxicated and attempts suicide could be held until he or she is detoxified, but after that brief period he or she should be released to do as one pleases.[42] At first glance this sounds reasonable: it seems to provide a clear cut-off point for intervention and would prohibit lengthy hospitalization solely as a means of preventing suicide. It seems to respect liberty while at the same time recognizing that some cannot exercise any liberty. Moreover, the criteria for distinguishing when we may intervene appear to be drawn in a clear manner including cases that few would dispute. Nevertheless, on inspection this move is caught in insuperable difficulties. Drugs and alcohol are not the only things that distort a person's view of one's life and circumstances. To believe that they are is false. Severe depression or schizophrenia can alter the process of reasoned deliberation as much as drug or drink. But this fact proves fatal to the move we are considering. If one still wishes to limit intervention to cases of intoxication, the rationale for doing so will be difficult to produce. It cannot now be that these are the only cases in which capacities for rational choice are impaired in reversible ways. Depression, for example, is eminently treatable with a variety of

195

biologically based therapies. If, however, the policy of intervention does remain limited to intervention only in cases of intoxication, one is committed to allowing thousands of lonely, depressed people like Mr. N to kill themselves even though their depression is very likely to respond to corrective treatment. This seems to me to be a telling objection to any such limitation.

Without such a limitation, however, this position collapses into a general analysis of the competency of the patient, which, as we saw, will require a judgment regarding the proposed suicide itself. To admit that we may intervene to help people like Mr. N is to ask us to judge more than inebriation. It is to ask us to judge their reasons for wishing to kill themselves. This, of course, puts us back where we started without any plausible answer from "new consensus" writers concerning when suicide is reasonable and when it is not.

Such a knowledge entails the belief that we know when it would be reasonable to conclude that a given life is not worth living. Furthermore, as policy such a standard would necessarily be a public standard for making the relevant determination concerning individual lives. It is to assume that we know when life is and is not "worth it," and thereby which lives should be protected and nourished by the rest of us. Instead of supporting and protecting all life, we should support those who aid in the termination of those lives that do not meet whatever criterion is set. Though the "new consensus" writers wanted to avoid just such a conclusion, it seems apparent that they cannot if they wish to offer any guidance on policy questions. Insofar as they wish to do so. They are involved in precisely this fundamental departure from our civic tradition that we have noted throughout this book.

The fundamental difficulties with the "new consensus" position can now be summarized. It started out wanting to modify the strong position regarding an individual's right to commit suicide endorsed by those such as Szaz or Hume. But whether it was making an argument about morality or about law and public policy is unclear. If it was the latter, then two alternatives presented themselves. First it could revert to the position, similar to Szaz's, *as policy* and then argue that *in actual fact* most cases of suicide or attempted suicide are moral wrongs. This turned out to be so unreasonable that a second move was often made: permit suicide intervention in some set of cases and protect the right of the individual to kill himself in other cases. Unfortunately this too seemed to fail because none of the available alternatives for discriminating among these classes of cases appeared to be plausible or promising as a policy for the great majority of suicide cases and, more seriously, because any public attempt to do so necessarily involves a public definition of a life not worth living and the difficulties attendant on any such judgment. Hence we must turn elsewhere if we seek an acceptable public resolution to the question of suicide and assisting in suicide. Paradoxically this will return us, in general, to the typical policies regarding suicide intervention and suicide assistance that already exist in most states.

A Nuanced Policy

With the collapse of the Szazian position and the "new consensus" variant, we are left with one realistic direction in which to pursue alternatives for public and professional practice. This direction is one that permits intervention by professionals with suicidal attempts or gestures solely on a showing that suicidal behavior is involved. This is, of course, the essential core of current mental health policy and I see no persuasive rationale for changing it. Even if, on some grounds, we conclude with Aristotle, that suicide is justified in some rare cases, it is abundantly clear that such cases will constitute no more than a very tiny fraction of the whole. On the contrary, the reality is that the vast majority of suicidal persons are like Mr. N sick, depressed human beings or like Mr. A. extremely ambivalent about what they really wish to do. Even assuming for the sake of argument that a very few suicides are justified, it clearly seems wrong to adopt a policy for the tiny fraction that ignores the real needs of the larger whole. To let many people kill or injure themselves unjustly to avoid a possible wrong to a very few is a poor trade-off even in terms of the consequentialist moral theory that must be adopted if suicide is to be justified at all.

Furthermore, this policy will actually work little hardship in those cases where the justification for permitting an individual to commit suicide is most compelling. Two points can be stressed in this regard. First, those who have firmly decided to kill themselves will not be very likely to engage in suicidal gestures or announcements of their intent which only call attention to their situation. The people who call attention to their suicide in these ways are disturbed persons who seek to manipulate others; rarely do they actually wish to die.[43] Moreover, the kinds of personality disorders which they manifest are hardly those we would wish to see in a perfectly rational choice for suicide. Secondly, those who really are rational enough and free from coercive pressures such that their choice might deserve respect by any reasonable "new consensus" standards, will not likely fail in the means once they have reasonably and courageously decided on the end itself. They will not be the people who take only enough sleeping pills to make themselves sick but far from a lethal dose, or shoot themselves in the shoulder instead of in the head. Those whose suicide would come under any reasonable standard of justified suicide will be competent enough to do the deed without being discovered and prevented or failing to complete it. Those who are likely to fail in the completion of a suicidal act will be those whose firmness in the choice or competence to so choose must be questioned. Of course it is precisely in these cases that intervention is most in order.

In short, this policy alternative will cause less possible injustice than any of the alternatives, even if we assume that there are rare cases of justified suicide. It does not sacrifice the lives and health of the vast number to the supposed freedom of the tiny fraction; nor does it actually interfere very much with the liberty of those who really have rational and well-thought-out desires of and means of killing themselves. Finally, it does not capitulate to the passions of the depressed and psychotic persons who most often want to kill themselves.

Conclusion

The problem of suicide has perplexed western thought since ancient times. The literature concerning it is vast and covers a wide range of disciplines and perspectives. From an abstract point of view, it raises central questions of philosophy and theology and has been recognized as a crucial problem for many moralists in both secular and theological terms. For various schools of psychiatry and psychotherapy, suicide has also been a fertile field for theoretical formulations and developments.

It is not disparaging to the theoretical importance of the topic if we conclude here that, from the point of view of policy, suicide is the easiest of the issues treated in this book. The overwhelming evidence is that suicidal persons are impaired, disturbed human beings who need help and love and care, not death. If they really wish to kill themselves, they will do so without the help of any supposed right to kill themselves. In fact, it is the very anomic society of isolated individuals, whose moral dialogue is dominated by talk of individual rights, that has brought these people to their point of despair.

At this point public policy cannot make life meaningful for those who have lost meaning. It cannot re-create the bonds of communal care that have been severed in countless ways for countless persons. For these, the suicidal person must look elsewhere: to family, neighborhood, friendship and religious community. But public policy can preserve the possibility of this reconstruction by giving these sources of meaning a space to work. For many they will reconstruct enough meaning to make life livable. For others life has become so filled with despair that no amount of love can make it bearable. These people will kill themselves. As a people we need not cloak that loss of meaning in the morally and politically powerful language of rights. Suicide is a symbol of loss, not hope and once cloaked in our most powerful civic language, that loss will surely grow and that language itself suffer.

CHAPTER SIX

Abortion

Introduction

Abortion is without question the most divisive issue in contemporary American political life. Few issues since the Civil War have touched off as bitter a national debate as the current dispute over abortion. Ironically, the bitterness and passion surrounding this issue have increased since the Supreme Court decreed a national policy of abortion on demand. This fact suggests the fundamental nature of the abortion question and the utter failure of the Supreme Court to articulate a proper basis for a national consensus regarding it. On other divisive issues, the Court has found the requisite means to articulate a national consensus; legally enforced segregation of the schools is a prime example. No political leader of any national or regional significance now defends a return to the era before *Brown v. Board of Education.* For all its extensive faults in judicial reasoning and policy scholarship, the result in *Brown,* namely, that children ought not to be assigned to schools solely because of race, was just. Even white southerners, whose immediate hostility was to be expected, came to see the justness of this result in what was, considering the history involved, a rather short time. The absence of any such cooling of passions in regards to abortion, in fact the deepening intransigence and political paralysis engendered by it, seem telling evidence that the Court failed to meet the rationale for constitutional review which its most sober defenders have always offered.[1]

Nonetheless, as it stands, the abortion question is somewhat different from the other issues of public policy discussed in this book. In the other cases that have concerned us, the presence of a human being about whom decisions must be made is a silently unchallenged assumption. One therefore starts with the tension between equality and liberty. As such, one decides if this person's equal worth as a person is no longer present, or where the tension between individual liberty and equal worth exists, one tries to decide where to strike the balance in this context; but one does not, except in the extreme case, doubt that the decision involves a human being about whom such awesome decisions must be made. The question is one of striking a balance among rights and among bearers of rights. The question of whether a bearer of rights exists rarely rise.

That very question, however, is of central importance in the proper consideration of abortion. Only if the human status of the fetus is granted, do we have a matter that ought to be a public concern at all. If it is not a human being: if, for example, it is the body tissue which feminists claim it to be, the disposing of it must be a private matter between the woman and her physician. Resolving the status of the fetus, therefore, seems to be a necessary precondition to the formulation of proper public policy on abortion.

Since this question differs materially from those that have concerned us so far in this book, we do not have the space to explore its many nuances. Nevertheless, for a consideration of public policy, a solution to the question of the humanity of the fetus is rather easily located. Though easy to locate, however, such a solution will require transcending the position of the Supreme Court and the patent absurdities on much proabortion rhetoric on the subject. To these matters we now turn our attention.

In its decision the Court initially claimed that it did not know whether the fetus was a being with human standing or not.[2] This admission might have led the judiciary to defer to legislative findings on the question. However, the Court further claimed that it did not need to answer the question because, in any case, the fetus was definitely not a person for constitutional purposes.[3] The speciousness of this maneuver is patent; most commentators, even those favorable to abortion on demand recognized this. The only precedent for such a separation between a human being and a constitutionally recognized person is slavery, where the humanity of the black person was admitted, but his or her constitutional standing denied. Such a precedent is not likely to find much favor today.

Only if this separation is made, however, will the Court's position be coherent. Without it, the Court is plainly sanctioning the killing of millions of unborn children merely because one of their parents does not want them. This result is scarcely intelligible to anyone raised in our moral and legal tradition. This point also seems to be admitted by most of the defenders of the Court's conclusion, who have generally attempted to supply the argument or arguments that are absent in the Court's discussion.[4]

Even accepting the Court's bifurcation of human being and person, its position regarding legal personhood will not stand. For practical purposes, the Court claims that a legal person comes into being at the point of viability, when the fetus has the potentiality to exist apart from the mother's womb. Then and only then are the states permitted to protect the unborn from the actions of the mother. Aside from the elusiveness of this magic point itself, viability is perhaps the weakest of all the available alternatives for marking the existence of a legally recognized person. Viability means nothing more than the move from a state in which this fetus is utterly dependent for his or her life on this specific woman to a state where most fetuses are dependent only on another human being, not necessarily one individual woman.

But such dependency and the burdens it imposes are not limited to the fetus, either in theory or reality. Usually, of course, someone else is available to assume care in cases of helpless dependency at either end of life—infancy or old age. It is useful, however, to ask ourselves about cases where this cannot or will not be done. For example would a person have a right to go away and leave an infant to starve, if no one else would assume care, asserting that his or her freedom was the paramount claim at stake? Or consider Siamese twins. Would we accept the plea of one twin for his or her freedom when detaching him or her from the mate would necessarily entail the death of the other? Would a nursing mother in a primitive area be justified in asserting the value of her freedom over the life of the infant when no other nursing mothers were available to assume care and the infant would starve without such food. It seems to me that the answer to these cases is obvious, especially in legal and policy terms.[5] If so, the Court's reliance on viability—that is, the supposed absence of one kind of dependency—to define legal personhood, fails.

The Human Status of the Human Fetus

Once the Supreme Court decision is set aside, we can confront directly the question of the fetus about to be aborted; from this confrontation, I believe, we can easily obtain the answer to our query about his or her human standing. One hears a good deal these days about the zygote, that uniquely endowed organism created by the union of sperm and ovum, which is putatively what is removed in an abortion. In practical terms however, the zygote is a red herring in the consideration of abortion. By the time the woman has ascertained that she is pregnant, and has had time to decide on and schedule an abortion, the being within her has progressed well beyond the zygote stage. In the properly developing pregnancy, the fetus about to be aborted will usually have human parentage, a unique human genetic code, human anatomical form and appearance, detectable brain activity, and a functioning circulatory system.[6] Late second trimester abortions, such as those necessary after diagnosis of a genetic abnormality in the fetus, destroy a being that has obtained virtually complete physiological development.[7] At this point it would seem relevant to ask: why should anyone have considered the fetus about to be aborted as anything other than an unborn human being, indistinguishable from one's slightly older siblings which the Court allows us to protect?

Once the relevance of this question is granted, it appears to be a simple matter to conclude that the intentional termination of a known pregnancy almost surely takes the life of a human being and as such should be restricted in conformity with other common and statutory laws restricting the taking of human life. Moreover, since the exact gestational age of any fetus cannot be known with absolute certainty, it would be a wise policy to extend this protection as far back as possible in pregnancy. Such a restriction would specify only that what is restricted is the intentional termination of a known pregnancy.

While the usefulness of such a conclusion for policy purposes seems obvious, it is open to two sorts of fundamental challenges. First, some people still wish to deny the humanity of the fetus by adding on to the biological basis noted above such other capacities as self-consciousness, sentience, or the presence of desires or interests which the fetus is not known to possess. While this move may successfully exclude the fetus from the human family, it also excludes newborn infants, profoundly retarded persons, senile, aged individuals, and comatose patients, even those in any of these classes on a temporary basis, as is the fetal condition only temporary.[8] At the policy level, such results seem to be compelling reasons for rejecting such maneuvers.

One interesting attempt to rescue this line of attack on the humanity of the fetus is contained in a recent discussion by Becker.[9] The essence of his argument is that human beings develop along a continuum that can be divided into two basic sections. The first is a process of biological development culminating in a morphologically complete organism. The second is a process of biological growth and psychological development culminating in the full grown adult. The first section is termed by Becker the *entry process* or the *becoming* stage. The successful completion of this becoming is considered to be a *sine qua non* for the existence of a human being. "The completion of the metamorphic phase of generative development is a necessary condition of the completion of the entry process—that is, the becoming/being boundary cannot be put any earlier than this."[10]

Despite a superficial plausibility, this position is both unclear and difficult to sustain. The unclarity comes from a confused use of morphological considerations to determine whether an entity is a human being or not. Even granting, as I have done above, the cogency of morphological considerations, Becker's position is confusing. At the outset he tells us that a human being is present:

> When its metamorphic like process is complete—that is when the relatively undifferentiated mass of the fertilized human ovum has developed into the pattern of differentiation characteristic of the organism it is genetically programmed to become.[11]

Unfortunately, this mixes two vastly different sorts of morphological arguments. Perhaps he means that a human being exists when a distinctively human morphology exists. Surely this will be when a comparative biologist could say with certainty that this is a human morphology and can only be such. However, this occurs much earlier in pregnancy than the point—approximately six months gestational age—endorsed by Becker as the beginning of the "human being."[12] Even granting Becker's view, that entry into the class of human beings is a process, the essential thrust of this interpretation would be substantially similar to mine and the policy implication would be arguably the same.

The second interpretation comports better with Becker's notion that the becoming/being boundary is crossed at about six months gestational age, but it is difficult to sustain an argument for it. On this view the process of morphological development must be complete for entry to have occurred. In this context Becker contends that the entry process is complete when 1) the gross anatomical form is complete, and 2) the inventory of histologically differentiated organs is complete. It is, however, difficult to find a cogent argument for either proposition, especially the second. The analogy is to the development of the butterfly from the pupa; but taken seriously, the analogy will not support this conclusion. The differentiation between butterfly and pupa will surely be when a trained observer can make a reasonable judgment that this is a butterfly. But it hardly seems plausible to say that such a judgment is not possible until a microscopic examination shows all organ systems complete.

I believe that the point is even clearer for the human fetus. It may be admitted that we need to distinguish between a formless mass of cells in the blastocystic stage and the presence of the "shape and general arrangement of the parts."[13] But that does not imply that we must have every organ histologically complete. For example, suppose that an infant is born with a dysfunctional heart but can be attached to a much improved artificial heart until his or her heart can be repaired. It seems strongly counterintuitive to say that here we have not a human being but only a human becoming, in Becker's terminology. One can go down the list of anatomical and physiological parts, and suppose them to be missing or incompletely formed in a neonate, requiring medical intervention at birth. To suppose that in any of these cases we do not have a human being only a human becoming seems so far out of touch with our common conceptual framework that I do not see how it can be plausibly maintained. Becker himself provides no reasons for doing so.

Once we grant that these are human beings, we cannot salvage Becker's morphological argument. We would need a different set of criteria focusing on an essential minimum of morphological and genetic characteristics such as I have noted above, which can be contained in a different interpretation of Becker's often loose phraseology about "patterns of differentiation characteristic of the organism." In short, we need to know the essential properties of a human being; these simply cannot be equated with complete morphological development. Any reasonable view regarding these essential properties would have policy implications similar to mine.

Putative Dangers of Restricting Abortions

The second line of attack seems more promising, at least to several recent commentators who have adopted it. Here the move is to skirt a proper confrontation with the fetal person by claiming that the abortion on demand position of the Court can be justified without any decision concerning the human standing of the fetus. For those who support the abortion on demand position of the Court, this line of argument seems appealing. If successful, it provides a rationale for the conclusion of the Court while sidestepping all the unsuccessful attempts to deny the humanity of the fetus which we have just noted. If this can be done, then the case for largely unrestricted access to abortion is compelling.

The arguments advanced for this conclusion are many but they can be grouped in four broad classes, each of which purports to show that legal restrictions on abortion should not be permitted. Generally, it is argued that restrictive abortion law is: 1) unenforceable as a policy, 2) largely harmful in its effects, 3) necessarily premised on impermissible religious grounds, or 4) an unjust attempt to force all women to live by a moral standard of self-giving behavior that is chosen only by a few persons. Though none of these arguments is adequate to the task for which they are employed, it behooves us to lay them to rest with some precision.

Unenforceable

One of the most common claims made by advocates of abortion on demand is that restrictive abortion laws do not actually prevent abortion. From this presumption, they conclude that such laws should not be enacted since widespread lapses in enforcement breed disrespect for the law in general and any attempt at enforcement will simply drive women to illegal and unsafe abortions. The crucial premise is the claim

that restrictive abortion laws only force individuals to find illegal sources of abortion.[14] The true abortion rate, it is said,
remains the same in either case.

Unfortunately, this argument cannot be saved by the facts.
Data available from many countries show that restrictive abortion law does in fact seriously affect the actual incidence of
abortion. In many parts of Eastern Europe, abortion laws were
substantially liberalized after World War II.[15] In every instance
the number of abortions rose sharply. In some countries abortion became a primary means of contraception, as it presently is
in some parts of the United States for some women.[16] It is very
unlikely that such a use of abortion would occur if access to it
were seriously restricted.

While these data surely cast doubt on the premise that a
restrictive abortion law is unenforceable, that premise is com-
pellingly rebutted by even better data from Britain and the
United States. In Britain before the passage of a very liberal
abortion law in 1967, there were about twenty-thousand abortions annually, both legal and illegal.[17] This rate was calculated
from the one figure that is hard to distort—the incident of
maternal deaths due to abortion. A British national survey
estimated the total at closer to thirty thousand abortions annually, a figure which is not substantially dissimilar for our purpose.[18] By the middle of the 1970s, the abortion rate in Britain
hovered around 110,000 abortions annually. What the unenforceability thesis must presuppose, therefore, is that around
eighty-thousand British women would have illegal abortions in
1974 when they and their slightly older cohorts did not do so in
1966. Such a conclusion is so completely counterintuitive and
unsupported by anything we know about human behavior that
we can safely reject it here.

In America the available data demonstrates the same conclusion. Syska, Hilgers, and O'Hare have recently developed a
model for estimating criminal abortions from maternal mortality.[19] Working from data that consciously overestimated the
incidence of criminal abortion in the prelegalization era, the
authors found a steep rise in the number of abortions after
abortion law was liberalized in favor of abortion on demand.

"With legalized abortion," they write, "there has been an exponential increase in the total number of abortions each year in the United States, in the range of 6 to 11-fold from the prelegalization era."[20] The facts are clear: legalizing abortion substantially increases the true incidence of abortion.

Once these facts become clear, the unenforceability argument loses its force completely. If many abortions will be prevented by legal restrictions, then the probability that some will be performed anyway hardly constitutes a good reason for refusing to prevent those killings that we can prevent, given a good case for restrictive abortion law on other grounds. The mere fact that most murders or most white-collar crime goes unpunished hardly offers grounds for repeal of the statutes in question.

Much the same can be said of the justice or fairness variant of this argument, wherein it is claimed that whatever abortions are prevented will be those sought by persons too poor, too uneducated, or too ill-situated to obtain an illegal one. This, it is argued, violates elementary standards of justice. Such a state of affairs may be unfair but it does not follow that the means of correcting such an unfairness is to repeal all restrictions on the practice in question. Other groups such as organized crime can act illegally almost at will. Yet such a fact provides no reason to repeal these laws and an even more compelling case for seeing that they are fairly enforced.

Grave Harms to Women

The harm argument rests on the same premise as the enforceability argument but it proceeds in a different and somewhat weaker fashion. In its simplest form, it claims that restrictive abortion laws drive women to quacks who kill, injure, or maim them. Given the fact that a legal prohibition of abortion will prevent many abortions, this argument must rest on a very dubious policy choice. Its advocates must prefer the health or possibly the life of a relatively few women over the lives of thousands of fetuses/persons who would be alive if given a chance. Conventional utilitarianism would not generate this

choice and it is very difficult to envision what alternative justification may be offered. Furthermore, following this same rationale, we should legalize any number of activities from the
use of drugs to prostitution where we may provide a safe environment for the practice of what would otherwise be an illegal
and potentially hazardous activity. Homicide or arson are dangerous acts for their perpetrators; many individuals die when
home-made bombs go off accidentally. The proposition that
this would constitute any plausible rationale for legalizing the
activity is absurd. If we really did accept the humanity of the
fetus, we would need to produce some extremely compelling
harms resulting from restrictive abortion laws to make this
argument work. Given the moral beliefs that lie at core of Western liberal regimes, I confess I cannot conceive what those
harms would be that would justify the continued killing of
thousands of small, weak, human beings.

Finally, it is sometimes alleged that restrictive abortion law
leads to unwanted and thereby abused children. The usual
assumption here seems to be that abortion is a way to prevent
the arrival of more abused children. Several things are wrong
with this argument. First, the vast majority of abused children
were wanted to begin with and abortion will do nothing to
prevent these cases of neglect and abuse. Child abuse seems to
stem from other intrafamilial and intrapsychic processes than
the mere presence of an originally unwanted and unplanned
birth. Secondly, there is no evidence that refused abortion leads
to an incidence of child abuse greater than what one would
expect from families similarly situated regarding many other
demographic variables. If so, then the claim advanced above
simply cannot be sustained, irrespective of the position taking
on the human status of the fetus. Furthermore, we must note
that if killing the child were an acceptable means of preventing
further child abuse, child abuse would disappear rapidly. This
suggestion is preposterous yet it highlights the fact that to
present a harm from abuse great enough to justify killing the
fetus, we must first silently deny his or her equal standing as a
human being.

Intrusion of Religion

By far the most widely publicized view of the relation of abortion to our civil polity and law is the claim that abortion is essentially a religious matter. On this account, legislative restrictions are both unconstitutional, because of the first amendment, and unjustified, because of the healthy respect for individual conscience that our society fosters and that is symbolized in the constitutional separation of church and state.[21]

Despite the attention given to this view of the abortion question by the popular media, the substantive argument offered in defense of it is the weakest of those that we shall examine. Its weaknesses are twofold: first, in its characterization of abortion as an issue and, second, in its implied understanding of the relation of religious bodies and spokesmen to public policy and legislative enactment.

The characterization of abortion as essentially a religious matter for constitutional purposes is simply wrong. The question of when the fetus/newborn becomes a human being entitled to protection is no more or less a religious question than were similar queries concerning Indians in the sixteenth century or blacks in the nineteenth century.[22] This is a conceptual matter that we may resolve in several different ways. We may appeal to evidence from genetics and embryology. We may draw analogies between the presence of brain activity in the fetus and the now widely accepted definition of death as the absence of brain activity. We may attempt to compare the fetus and the neonate. Ultimately, of course, we will have to adopt a coherent concept of "humanness" and apply that to the fetus. The argument advanced above, for example, made no reference to sectarian religious beliefs whatsoever. It did appeal to certain moral convictions that are fundamental in our civilization, but these will be part of any statutory enactment; homicide law is a case in point. In theory, therefore, the issue is in no politically relevant sense a matter that impermissibly mixes the realms of church and state.

The abortion issue does involve deeply held, sometimes

212

intractable, beliefs. But this is true on almost any matter of judicial or legislative activity. Consider the questions of slavery and desegregation. Are we to assume that because there were intractable, religiously justified beliefs concerning equality, inequality, and personality involved in this debate, that courts and legislatures should never have taken up the question? Once stated clearly, the claim involved here looks preposterous.

The second problem with this characterization of the abortion question is the way in which its proponents are forced to stretch the definition of the "essentially religious character" of a public issue. One proponent of this position, Frederick Jaffe, has written:

A belief could be distinguished as primarily religious by such criteria as the following: (1) it is part of the doctrine of religious groups; (2) it is legitimated in religious and transcendental terms; (3) its principal exponents are associated with religious groups as are the majority of its adherents; (4) individuals are formally taught the belief mainly through religious institutions; (5) the principal organizations supporting legislation embodying the belief are either religious institutions or closely allied organizations that draw a large part of their funds, cadres, constituency and advocacy networks from religious groups; and (6) advocacy for the belief is dominated by religious references and symbols.[23]

If this view were accepted, much of the legislative activism that liberals have admired would be impermissibly tainted with religious bias. For example, any dispassionate analysis of either the antislavery or the desegregation movements would easily demonstrate their religious character under these criteria. Jaffe might admit this and still maintain that while many legislative enactments involve deeply held, quasi-religious beliefs, we should only enact those on which their exists what he terms an "overwhelming consensus."

Unfortunately, no such consensus exists on a wide range of public issues that have nevertheless been quite properly seen as fit subjects for judicial or legislative involvement. Divorce is one obvious example, desegregation is another. Reverend Martin Luther King's march on Washington in 1963 could easily have been duplicated in reverse in Mobile or Birmingham with any number of fundamentalist preachers behind the podium. It appears that we are being told that every piece of civil rights legislation enacted in the past quarter century is impermissibly tainted with the religious opinions of only some citizens, not an overwhelming majority. The same can be said of divorce law, which in most states is deeply offensive to the sensibilities of orthodox Catholics, or autopsy law which is similarly offensive to orthodox Jews. Once applied across the spectrum of state and federal American law, Jaffe's position very rapidly loses any semblance of plausibility.

Intrusion of Moralism

Of the attempts to fill in the gaps in the Supreme Court decision, none is more interesting than that which claims that restrictive abortion law is a serious departure from our moral and legal traditions regarding the obligations of persons to save the lives of others. Though advanced from several sources, the claim is essentially the same: pre-*Roe* policies in most states required women to undertake essentially good Samaritan behavior toward the fetus.[24] That is, they required the woman to allow her body to be used to save the life of the fetus, a significant burden which she was required to bear. It is further alleged that common law has not traditionally required such behavior of people, even where life was at stake.[25] Generally, at common law, people are free to be bad Samaritans without fear at least of criminal sanctions. Such behavior may have been immoral but the only punishment was that imposed by a guilty conscience. It is concluded, therefore, that restrictive abortion law is an unjust imposition on the woman that can not be squared with our legal and political tradition.

The attractiveness of this position is obvious. If it can be successfully maintained, it will provide a rationale for abortions on demand and a justification for the Supreme Court's use of the elusive point of viability as the point at which the state may begin to prohibit abortion. Moreover this position appears to be

214

grounded in perceptions regarding the obligations of persons to perform heroic or saintly deeds which have intuitive appeal, well-known moral arguments on their behalf, and a common law tradition behind them. It is not difficult, therefore to discern why such a view has become popular with defenders of the abortion on demand position.

Unfortunately, this move fails without the addition of a hidden premise denying the humanity of the fetus. Common law usually does not require a person to be a good Samaritan. If I fail to rescue a drowning person when I could have done so, I will suffer no legal retribution. It is also arguable that when the victim is a complete stranger to me, when I have no prior relationship with the victim, I have no moral obligation to engage in good Samaritan behavior toward him or her. In neither case, of course, may I actually kill the person, but for the sake of argument, we will set this line of inquiry aside. Even if these general observations concerning the common law are granted, however, they seem to break down in cases most closely similar to those of a mother and an unborn child.

Consider again an infant born with an immune deficiency requiring it to have nursing mother's milk to survive, at least for a period in early infancy. It seems clear that the mother would have neither a moral nor a legal right to place the value of her freedom above the value of the life of her child, act accordingly, and let the child starve. The same conclusion seems to follow in other situations in which one person is utterly dependent on another for his or her continued existence, especially if the duration of the burden imposed is finite, as it is in pregnancy. In such situations neither our moral nor our legal traditions provide any support for the notion that one may opt out of such a relationship at one's choosing, preferring one's freedom over the life of the other.

The similarity of these cases to the situation of the fetus is obvious. In fact, the burden of caring for the total needs of the nursing infant is likely to be greater than that attending pregnancy, and the restrictions on the woman's mobility more severe. At least in the first six months of pregnancy, most women can move about quite as much as they wish and hold down demanding full-time jobs without endangering the life of the unborn child. Nursing mothers are usually confined to a much closer proximity to the child. This similarity is even true in an unplanned pregnancy. Consider our infant again. The mother in this instance surely did not plan on having such a child. But once the child is in her care, it seems both morally and legally proper to say that she has no right to relinquish such care if the infant will die without it.

One way out of these difficulties has been to focus on the specific physical burdens of pregnancy. These cannot be assumed by others, as can normal parental duties for unwanted children. Further, it is alleged that the common law views such burdens with special wariness in distinction from other burdens of care, such as financial support which the law places on parents who nevertheless want no part of any relationship with the child. This move may work to distinguish the normal situation of an unwanted infant from that of an unwanted pregnancy. The parent can always give the child up for adoption. But it is not successful against the cases I have presented, because these, like pregnancy, impose burdens which cannot be handed over to someone else. What is required is a demonstration that the physical burdens of pregnancy are greater than the burdens imposed in caring for an infant or anyone else who requires care where no alternatives are available. I simply do not know how this demonstration could be made successfully.

We must also note that, even if this argument were successful, it would only justify permitting abortion in those cases of completely unplanned and unwanted pregnancy. Even the law on good samaritan behavior typically does not allow a person who has started to save the life of someone to stop halfway through the act. If I am pulling a drowning person to shore, I may not simply stop halfway to shore and let the person drown.

But these observations suggest that only in cases of true contraceptive failure or forcible intercourse would this analysis, based on good samaritanism and the law, be successful. We only note in passing that the available data clearly demonstrate that many women are now using abortion as a primary means of contraception, or are using demonstrably ineffective means of contraception. Even if the above argument were granted, it would not reach their cases at all.

As the above analysis shows, the only way to make this whole argument successful is to silently deny the equal status of the fetus as a human being similar to the child. But once this is done, the attractiveness of this argument vanishes. It becomes little more than a restatement of one of the many reasons which a woman may give for wishing to remove herself from a relationship with the fetus. The apparent initial advantage of avoiding the question of the humanity of the fetus has disappeared.

The results of our discussion so far seem obvious. An acceptable resolution to the abortion issue, even in policy terms, requires resolving the question of the fetus. No move to avoid this question has proven successful. Confronting this question directly, however, we saw that by at least the time in pregnancy when most abortions are performed, the fetus is patently human. Abortions later in pregnancy, such as those following the required time necessary for prenatal genetic diagnosis, destroy beings who have acquired nearly complete physiological development.

The Emerging Public Policy

Sound public policy cannot ignore these observations. Taken together, they point to the necessity of rejecting the Supreme Court decision as the basis for public policy regarding abortion. The abortion on demand position of the Court required adoption of the proposition that until viability the fetus was not a human being in any politically or legally decisive sense. This view, we discovered, is untenable on several grounds. Having said this, however, implies nothing regarding the public policy that ought to replace our current practices. Pre-*Roe* practice was implicitly based on a recognition of the equal standing of both the fetus and the mother. Abortion was allowed in circumstances in which it was deemed impossible to give effect to the proper rights of both parties. But as yet we have said nothing of the stringency or leniency with which these circumstances are to be defined and whether they must be defined in a uniform manner across the nation or whether they may justly reflect the variations in opinion among the citizens of the various states. In forming a public policy on abortion, these are matters that must be resolved. But nothing that we have said as yet suggests the specific terms of any such resolution.

The Human Life Bill

To date three approaches have been advanced to surmount the Court's decision and move forward with more restrictions on the practice of abortion than are currently allowed. The first of these is the Human Life Bill sponsored by Senator Helms and Representative Hyde. This bill would:

1. putatively define the fetus as a human being from conception onward (a question on which the Court confessed its ignorance);
2. grant the fetus constitutional standing as a person (which the Court explicitly refused to do);
3. place the statute beyond the reach of the federal judiciary.[26]

The fundamental problem with the HLB is that it attempts to resolve a matter of constitutional right by purely statutory means. The willingness of antiabortionists to do this is readily understandable. They reject the Court's constitutional interpretation and as such they are loathe to admit it even to have it overturned. Unfortunately, it is not possible to ignore what the Court has done and thus the HLB is seriously defective. Congress surely does have the power to enter a legislative finding on point the first point. But without the addition of the second point, no measures actually restricting abortion will withstand scrutiny. At this point, however, the Human Life Bill proposes that Congress overturn by legislative enactment a clear constitutional holding of the Court. It is doubtful whether Congress has this power and it is more unlikely that the Court would acquiesce very readily in the exercise of any such power by Congress. This is different than the question of whether Congress has the power to restrict the jurisdiction of the federal courts, including the Supreme Court, in substantive ways by excluding certain matters, such as abortion and capital punishment, from judicial review. I believe that the only cogent reading of article three of the constitution will lead to an affirmation of such a power as asserted in section three of the HLB and a wide body of case law and scholarly opinion can be cited in its support. In any event, the attempt to achieve such a feat would result in a prolonged constitutional debate that might substantially detract from the actual goal of finding an appropriate means to transcend the abortion practices countenanced by the Court.

Even in more practical terms, the HLB is far from an optimal policy. Even granting the constitutionality of what is proposed under section three, namely, that the federal courts cannot review the legislation, their intimate involvement with the matter is certain. The HLB does not propose to repeal the rights which the Court found to be decisive in *Roe*—the woman's right of private reproductive choice. At most the HLB can be said to reassert a second right, the unborn child's constitutional right to life. When these rights conflict, someone must strike a balance between them, either in specific cases or in a range of such cases. It seems highly likely that such a balance will be struck by the federal courts, the usual place where a balance among competing constitutional rights is struck. Given the almost unrelenting hostility of the federal judiciary to the interests of the unborn in recent years, this is an odd place for anyone concerned with one's or her welfare to seek a balance that will be as protective as possible of the right of the unborn to life.

Constitutional Amendment Proposals:

Given the difficulties of the HLB, it appears to be a simple matter to conclude that we should enact some form of constitutional amendment that provides positive protection for the unborn. Several versions of such an amendment have been proposed; the most well known one is as follows:

> Section 1. With respect to the right to life, the word *person*
>   as used in this article and in the fifth and four-

teenth articles of amendment to the Constitution of the United States, applies to all human
beings, including their unborn offspring at every stage of their biological development, irrespective of age, health, function, or condition
of dependency.

Section 2. This article shall not apply in an emergency
when a reasonable medical certainty exists that
continuation of the pregnancy will cause the
death of the mother.

Section 3. Congress and the several states shall have power to enforce this article by appropriate legislation within their respective jurisdictions.[27]

At first glance this seems to be all we need. The unborn
child is given full constitutional status and the civic standing
that goes with it. An exception is made that no one disputes,
that can be defined with precision, and that will not expand
indefinitely in the direction of abortion on demand. On closer
inspection, however, serious problems emerge.

The first problem is purely political. There is nowhere near
the legislative support necessary to enact such a restrictive position on abortion. Hence it is argued that some less restrictive
amendment should be supported.[28] Political feasibility is not
within the scope of this book. What lies behind this concern,
however, is surely worthy of analysis.

Why is it that such an amendment would be difficult to
pass? It seems clear that on moral grounds many people would
find such an amendment too restrictive. It may prevent some
abortions whose case is, on balance, too compelling to dismiss.
Consider this actual case: A twelve-year-old severely retarded
girl with an IQ below 50 is raped in a school gym by three older
boys. The girl, though terrified of what has happened, had
little understanding of what had been done to her; nor did she
understand much about her resulting pregnancy. I submit that
for many persons there is a strongly held intuition concerning
the propriety of abortion here, even accepting the humanity of
the fetus. Such a considered judgment is at least as strong as
that held by those who seek the legal protection of the fetus

from the moment of conception onward. Yet the proposed amendment would not permit abortion in such a case, unless we could show that this girl's life is in danger from pregnancy. However, it seems clear that the conviction concerning the propriety of abortion here has little to do with any supposed risk to the life of the girl. She has been dealt a grave injustice. Forcing her to carry to term a pregnancy she can barely understand and cannot know the meaning of, strikes many as morally insensitive at best. This, of course, is a disputed conclusion. Nevertheless, it clearly seems to reflect at least as much moral sensitivity and intuitive strength as do the premises of the argument that may be advanced against it. It seems to me, therefore, that, at the very least, a legislature ought to be permitted to choose to reflect such a moral choice in its statutory regulations, since it presents a quite complex set of factual and policy issues.

The proposed amendment, however, would not permit such a legislative choice. In this it is considerably stricter than the abortion funding restrictions and substantially more rigorous than the law of many states before the Supreme Court decision. For example, by the early 1970s better than a dozen states had adopted the model abortion statute found in the American Law Institute's *Model Penal Code* (Proposed Draft, 1962) section 203.3. This provided that abortion was permitted whenever the pregnancy would threaten the life or health, including mental health, of the mother; where the pregnancy was the result of forced intercourse; or where the fetus would likely be born handicapped.

Finally, it is more restrictive than the considered moral beliefs of many otherwise morally sensitive individuals—who are still sympathetic to restrictive abortion legislation. One might assert that a case such as that of the young girl mentioned above is so rare that it ought not become the basis of public policy. Surely, if this amendment saved hundreds of thousands of lives, the hardship inflicted in this one case might be justified nonetheless. This point is important. It is patterned on the old adage that "hard cases make bad law," and it employs a form of reasoning widely used to shape public policies. Moreover, it can be justified on either utilitarian or modified

221

deontological grounds. Considered closely, however, it is unsuccessful on two grounds.

First, one would need to show that a legislative body, if given a chance, could not draft a statute that would only allow for exceptions in cases similar to this one. Without this showing it could still quite reasonably be maintained that allowing a few precisely drawn exceptions would not logically lead to opening the door to mass numbers of abortions. Unless it could be shown that we are incapable of keeping such a door closed, this argument will lose plausibility rapidly. Moreover, experience with the abortion funding amendments and with abortion law in the states before 1973 suggests that it would be very difficult to demonstrate the impossibility of drafting the appropriate statute. For example, if one wanted to include a psychiatric justification for abortion and still not open the door to abortion on demand, as happened under the ALI proposal, one may stipulate that, to qualify for abortion on grounds of mental health, one would have to have been in outpatient psychiatric care for nine months before abortion or within the last year one would have to have been treated as an inpatient in a psychiatric service for at least fifteen continuous days. This would weed out those merely seeking abortion from those with underlying psychopathology that might be exacerbated by pregnancy.

The rarity of such a case must be taken into account in judging the role it should play in our policy deliberations. A second sort of case we must consider is not rare at all: the use of the IUD as a contraceptive. It seems to me that the widespread use of the IUD, even by those who are sympathetic to the case against abortion, suggests that many otherwise well-informed persons see no incompatibility between the use of an admittedly abortifacient contraceptive device and opposition to the moral propriety of abortion in many cases.

Again, this is a conclusion that is disputed. The point is not to resolve that dispute here. What I maintain is that many conscientious individuals find nothing morally inappropriate with the IUD. Here, as in the case of rape, it seems clearly insensitive to rule out from the start the possibility that a legislature might find that their moral intuitions and the justifications that might be advanced for them were of sufficient strength and persuasiveness to be written into law, even a very restrictive abortion law.

It appears, therefore, that we need only amend this proposal to include such cases as exceptions. However, this is likely to be much more difficult than may be supposed at the outset. First, there will be difficult problems of drafting the language of any amendment in such a manner as to include precisely those abortions one wishes and exclude all the rest. Once one starts making exceptions to the proposed statute, one must exercise great care to avoid having the exceptions destroy the force of the general rule. It is not likely to be very easy to codify the permissible instances of abortion. Consider rape, for example. Do we wish to include all pregnancies due to rape or just some? Defining a subclass of rape-induced pregnancies would be extremely problematic as a matter of morality and probably impossible to codify as well. Yet allowing anyone who claims to have been raped to procure abortion thereby would surely destroy the force of any general rule against abortion.

This problem is difficult, but it may not be insoluble, as the debate over funding restrictions suggests. Until recent years congressional restrictions on abortion funding provided funding for abortion in cases where the rape or incest had been reported to a law enforcement agency or public health service clinic within seventy-two hours of its occurence. This provided a means of establishing that forced intercourse had occurred, and enabled funding agencies to refuse funding in cases where forced intercourse was claimed merely to obtain funding for abortion. Nevertheless, any solution is likely to involve extensive and delicately nuanced statutory language. At this point, however, it seems to me that the feasibility of this as a constitutional amendment becomes highly dubious. What started out as a simple amendment prohibiting abortion has become an extensive text resembling much more a state criminal statute than a constitutional provision.[29]

The search for a morally sensitive amendment has led to a

difficult impass. The only way in which an acceptable amendment can be written is to employ the constitution in a manner foreign to its history or the intentions of the founders. Drafting an acceptable amendment would, in effect, require us to incorporate a criminal statute into the constitution. Aside from the uneasiness with which such a development would be viewed, it has two fundamental problems. First, it badly confuses the purposes of constitutional and statutory law; secondly, it confuses the function of federal as opposed to state law.

Constitutions define the essence of political regimes. They establish the structures of governance, and the means of enacting laws and effectuating their enforcement.[30] They establish the fundamental means by which the conflicts inherent in communal life can be arbitrated. In a federal system constitutions divide the political whole and assign responsibility to the various parts. They give us some idea of who must perform what functions of government. Fire protection and law enforcement, for example, are still generally matters of local responsibility, while interstate commerce regulations are not, touching as they do on the interests of more than one state. Constitutions thus define the political whole in very broad strokes. They set out the parameters and leave the details to be worked out by the people and their leaders in new circumstances. But they do not define every situation and decide every matter of political governance and public policy. The minutiae of politics simply cannot be put into constitutional texts for the very reason that so many special interest groups want to see them so placed; the regime defining character of constitutional language necessitates a permanence not granted to simple statutory enactments. It is this permanence which renders unwise and impossible the inclusion of the details of governance and the nuances of statutory regulation. Of those details that can be seen, change is so likely that the needed flexibility would be severely compromised by inclusion in the constitution; the vast number of unseen problems could not be included at all. For example, in the debate over the tenth amendment, reserving undelegated powers to the people or the states, Tucker of South Carolina sought

224

to amend the draft to include the word *expressly* delegated. Such a wording would have profoundly altered the constitutional history of America. No less a figure than Madison objected; he said "it was impossible to confine a government to the exercise of express powers; there must necessarily be admitted powers by implication unless the constitution descend to recount every minutiae."[31]

We do not want our constitution to reflect the temporary needs or passions of the many or the fluctuating knowledge of contemporary science. Nor do we wish it to reflect highly nuanced moral choices that are open to great change. Consider the question of abortion itself. At the time of the American founding, what little statutory law existed on abortion would have been deeply offensive to devout prolife advocates. These statutes generally permitted abortion up to the time of "quickening," when the mother could feel the fetus move. These laws had a complex background in the common law but at least part of their *raison d'être* was a belief, ultimately derived from Aristotle, which held that the soul did not enter the body until the mother felt the fetus move.[32] This was the decisive point when the fetus became a person with a human soul. That we now consider such a view completely mistaken only underscores the difficulties that would attend any attempt to force constitutional texts to reflect such supposedly scientific beliefs.

The second problem here is the matter of federalism. To achieve the protection of the fetus in a responsible fashion, we would need to write into the constitution a homicide statute. In so doing we would make a certain type of homicide a federal constitutional violation, in distinction from every other subtype of homicide or manslaughter which are wholly covered by state criminal law. In every other analogous category, such as murder, manslaughter, and child abuse, the legal protections afforded citizens are all found in state codes, not federal law and certainly not the constitution. These codes differ greatly, in both the definitions of the offense covered and the penalties attached. There are even more profound differences in the enumeration of mitigating or excusing circumstances in both statutory and common law. In some American jurisdictions a person will be charged with murder for what elsewhere might be ruled justified self-defense homicide.[33]

Yet for all the unfairness that seems to result from these differences, we still leave homicide law to the states, trusting in the good sense of the legislative and executive branches of state government to remedy these inequities. The alternative would be to give up federalism at its most pervasive and central point—the right of states to enact their own civil and criminal laws. To compromise federalism at this point is to give up a liberty cherished by Americans and written into their national compact from the very beginning, something that is at least as much a part of their regime as is any principle to which those supporting a constitutional solution to the abortion question might appeal.[34]

The problems with amendments such as noted above are inherent in the attempt to utilize the constitution for purposes foreign to its end and tradition. Of course, if making abortion a federal and constitutional matter were the only way to prevent the millions of deaths involved, then it seems clear that we would be remiss in not pursuing this course, even given the problems we have outlined. This is a course which no morally concerned person could avoid.

However, it is not the only way to transcend the existing state of affairs in which the Supreme Court has made abortion on demand a constitutional right and completely negated any civic standing for the fetus. The alternative means of moving away from the Supreme Court's ruling in *Roe* is to return the question of abortion and its proper social regulation to the people and their elected representatives in the various states. From the purely practical point of view this alternative has much to recommend it. The people of each state would be free to adopt detailed, nuanced abortion legislation that reflected the moral convictions of the citizens of the state as well as the inherent complexities involved in some cases of abortion.

Appropriate exceptions to any general rule could be included in as detailed and nuanced a fashion as necessary. Committee review could be included, as is the practice in Canada;

waiting periods could be mandated as means to ensure a stable, well-thought-through desire for abortion. The constitution would not be employed for the purposes of enacting a homicide statute as would the alternative.

This much said, we must still confront the central argument against such an amendment, one heard from both sides of the abortion controversy. Antiabortionist Charles Rice puts it in a powerful form:

> The states' right amendment would write into the constitution the totalitarian idea that innocent human beings hold their lives at the discretion of legislative majorities. For this reason, the amendment is morally and intellectually bankrupt. It would be like fighting World War II for the principle that each locality in Germany should have the right to decide its own death camp. Innocent life would become a subject of political negotiation and bartering, just like a highway or school appropriation. The amendment, moreover, would endanger, in addition to the unborn, the lives of the senile, the retarded and other vulnerable classes through its implication that there is a power but not a duty to protect life at whatever stage.[35]

Excusing his rhetoric, Rice's argument is important. Certainly it appears that the states' rights amendment regarding abortion employs the same dubious logic as did the appeals to states' rights in defense of slavery, segregation, and other evils. Is not this appeal to state regulation as offensive, both morally and politically, as was a similar appeal by Senator Stephen Douglas in his debates with Lincoln? Does not this amendment likewise permit a legislative majority to endorse or allow the worst evils, such as murder of the unborn, who are admitted to be human beings? The sensitivity of this result appears difficult to defend, especially considering the expressed desire to offer legal protection to unborn persons.

Despite appearances, this argument is deeply flawed. To be for the rights of state legislatures to set their own laws is not *ipso facto* to be for the evils that might be done by a legislatively constituted majority. That is a perennial problem of democratic regimes; and it does not go away by appealing to a constitutional restriction. Need we be reminded that slavery once enjoyed constitutional status and could again were it not for the good sense of the people. If an active majority wishes something, such as prohibition, it can be achieved even if the constitution needs to be amended to accomplish it.[36]

Therefore, the claim that a states' rights amendment on abortion would permit the people to decide to legalize what are believed to be grossly immoral activities is true. But that truth is coeval with democratic regimes. To argue against such a situation is to transcend the limits of democratic rule itself in search of a very different polity. This is a proposition that is not advanced by Rice and does not appear to be at issue here.

In this regard the abortion question is fundamentally dissimilar from the slavery question with which antiabortionists constantly wish to compare it. Of course, in both cases the Supreme Court's egregious departure from sound constitutional interpretation forced a resolution at the national level. However, slavery was a relatively simple issue to resolve. There were no conceivably just reasons to continue it in any special case. It could be ended, as it was, by a short constitutional amendment. A proper resolution of the abortion question will not be found in that fashion. There are too many cases in which abortion is clearly or arguably just to permit such a resolution as would be acceptable in a constitutional provision. Viewed in this light, a states' rights amendment is the only path by which the injustice of post-*Roe* practice can be transcended in a manner consistent with justice itself, as well as with the special requirement of a federal republic which leaves criminal law in the hands of the states.

Even the protection afforded by Rice's cherished constitutional solution may be more illusory than real unless we move to a full national homicide law. Under the uniform proposal, the states are not required to adopt strict abortion laws. If they refused to do so, the only recourse for those concerned to protect the unborn would be a suit for the unborn alleging the deprivation of a constitutional right. At that point the matter reverts to the federal courts to strike a balance between the constitutional rights of the woman and her alleged interests in health and freedom and the right to life of the unborn. Given the willingness of the courts to defend abortion on demand, it takes little imagination to know where that balance is likely to be struck in difficult, borderline cases.

Of course, with the adoption of the uniform national proposal, we are likely to have substantially more restrictions on abortion than we have today. It is difficult to conceive of any court striking a balance in favor of abortion on demand if the fetus is declared to be a person for constitutional purposes. Nonetheless, the problem of court adjudication remains; the likelihood that the courts would permit of some exceptions beyond the saving of a mother's life surely opens the door to other exceptions. Such a result would hardly be acceptable to hard core antiabortionists such as Rice. The only alternative is to give up legal federalism altogether and adopt a national homicide statute. Under such a statute, Congress could prohibit anything it wishes to prohibit and allow abortion in any circumstance it desired. As noted above this would be a radical revision of the American constitutional framework of republican federalism, in effect throwing the baby out with the bathwater. It also might not withstand constitutional challenge itself. The tenth amendment expressly reserves to the states and the people those powers that were not delegated to the national government. Given the historic legal framework of the American regime, it is hard to conceive of any assumption of federal power more alien to the intentions or the desires of the founders than would be a national homicide statute.

Even under such a statute, Congress would not be compelled to protect the unborn. Their lives like ours would be protected only to the extent that the guardians of political power chose to do so. The unborn would have to trust the virtue and good sense of legislative office holders and appointees as we all must. This of course is a problem of political rule itself for which neither Rice nor anyone else has found a perfect solution compatible with the premises of democratic regimes.

Such a national homicide statute may be the only way to salvage the uniform amendment which is the goal of many antiabortionists like Rice. Other alternatives exist, however, for meeting the serious objections to a states rights proposal advanced by Rice and others. Perhaps the most promising move to date is the amendment submitted by Senator Hatch which reads:

Section 1. The right to an abortion is not secured by this constitution.

Section 2. Congress and the states shall have concurrent power to pass legislation giving force to this amendment.[37]

The Hatch proposal has two features that distinguish it from previous proposed amendments that would return the matter of abortion to the states for regulation. First it states clearly that abortion is not a matter of constitutional right. It thus represents a complete break with the dubious constitutional and jurisprudential thinking that permeates *Roe.* As we have suggested, this is a necessary precondition for shaping proper public policy in this area.

The most significant advance over previous drafts, however, is contained in the wording of section two. It establishes the concurrent power of Congress and the states to regulate abortion. Essentially this permits congress to establish some minimum national floor of protection for the fetus. The states would then be permitted to fill in the details and nuances of the policy and deal with the tough cases in accordance with the wishes of the citizens of their own states. For example, congress could adopt as a minimum the previous model bill of the American Law Institute. It provided for abortion in cases of rape or incest, when the fetus would be born with handicaps, or where the life, health or mental health of the mother was at risk. The ALI proposal led to virtual abortion on demand in some situations, especially when "mental health" was included. A state might eliminate such a provision or tighten the criteria necessary to certify it to prevent the automatic certification of anyone seeking abortion. This might be accomplished by requiring that the woman has been in regular psychotherapy, or that she has been admitted for inpatient psychiatric care for a specified duration during the preceding year.

It seems to me that this feature of the Hatch proposal meets all the objections against a constitutional amendment regarding abortion that can be met within the confines of democratic federalism. It does not require writing into the constitution an inappropriate criminal code, nor does it even require that the operative sanctions against abortion be a matter of federal law. It permits the people of the states to write abortion law in accordance with their own consciences yet provides a means by which the unborn will not be left utterly unprotected by any state—provided congress acts. In this regard, it offers some barrier to the creation of complete havens where abortion on demand would still flourish.

What it cannot do is place the life of the unborn utterly beyond the reach of the shifting views of legislative majorities. That is something which law in democratic regimes cannot do for any class of human beings. Essentially we are all at the mercy of such majorities. If a man enters my office right now and kills me he will be punished. We hope that the knowledge of that punishment deters my enemies from such action. But a legislative majority could change that law anytime it wished, making my existence substantially more precarious. This is a problem of democracy itself, namely, the necessity of placing our trust in citizens and leaders who are imperfectly wise, virtuous, just, and compassionate. But the answer for this problem is not to be found in the context of democratic regimes themselves and as such it goes beyond the scope of this book and the context of the discussion of abortion policy in our regime as well.

Conclusion

Our foray into the web of abortion policy has necessarily been rather brief. On some of the issues noted here, whole volumes have been written. Those who wish may delve further; the notes to this chapter provide references to much additional literature. We have at least sketched the outline of what seems to be a responsible public approach to abortion, one which requires none of the dubious jurisprudence or logical failures of the Supreme Court decision, or of its defenders. Moreover, our solution still permits citizens of various states to retain a substantial measure of authority to regulate this practice in accordance with their conscientious choices regarding the respective rights of the mother and child. In this regard, I believe that the policy advanced in this chapter substantially enhances the most cherished right available to citizens in any regime: the right to govern themselves.

CHAPTER SEVEN

From Policy to Practice

Introduction

In the four preceding chapters of this book, we examined how the central conviction of the equal worth of all human lives should work out in some core issues of contemporary medical policy. If I am right, public policy cannot endorse quality-of-life concepts, such as a "life not worth living," that strike at the foundation of a liberal polity. Not only do such concepts entail a fundamental break with our organizing principles; they are so vaguely worded and so elastic in their extension that they must lead to enormous disparities in practice.

Yet these are problems of public and medical policy formalized in law and hospital rules. Such considerations are important insofar as they set the context and establish the acceptable limits of policy. But these limits do not inform us how to resolve properly specific cases with unique nuances and complications. They do not specify if or when care may be withheld or withdrawn in a given case. Indeed, most great political theorists of the Western tradition have noted the limited capacity of law

233

and policy to guide human action.[1] So far we have only seen that law and policy cannot adopt quality-of-life standards to guide and legitimate these decisions. In this chapter we will prescind from the policy concerns that have structured the previous discussion, and examine how the conclusions we have reached might be applied in the context of actual medical practice. Would these conclusions substantially alter medical practice and distort the possibilities for humane care? If so, should practice therefore depart substantially from law and policy? If not, then what is the range of choice within which practice must take place?

This examination is necessary to complete our task for two reasons. First, a most serious criticism that might be brought against the policy sketched here is that it so completely varies from contemporary practice that it cannot possibly serve to guide clinical decisions or inform the deliberations of hospital committees. Even more: some might hold that, when contemporary practice diverges from my suggestions, it does so to provide more just and humane treatment of patients. If this were true, my proposals would tend to increase human suffering and misery; any policy that would force this on us cannot be correct. Secondly, we must be very clear about how far and in what way the conclusions reached earlier relate to clinical practice and personal choice. Otherwise, these conclusions remain abstractions, futile in meeting the most difficult questions of practical choice.

Data for Decision Making

The rhetoric of some medical and nonmedical spokesmen implies that a policy which would exclude the concept of a "life not worth living" is so divorced from actual practice that it can provide no guidance for clinical decisions. At first glance this would seem to be irrelevant to our task: the mere fact that most people do something surely does not establish any conclusions regarding its morality. In theory, of course, this is true. The acceptance of abortion on demand, for example, does not justify the practice. Nevertheless, if one intends to establish a

234

framework for actual choice, one must at least heed the manner in which people actually choose. A policy that presents something as choiceworthy or required which few regard as such either will be ignored or will entail despotic acts to enforce its choice.

This point must be carefully understood. I do not claim that policy must be so constructed as to legitimate whatever is desired as practice. Rather, the capacity of policy to guide practice entails two points: first, policy must be nuanced enough to adequately address the realities necessarily confronted in practice, without sacrificing its essential purpose; secondly, policy must call our attention to values and ways of acting that people can, on reflection, come to accept. To be sure, policy may impose solutions that not everyone agrees with. But at the very least, it should articulate solutions that most reasonable people will find plausible enough to obey.

Therefore, the questions that are essential to our inquiry are whether or not contemporary practice is so wedded to quality-of-life considerations that excluding them would either lead practitioners to ignore the policy or encourage inhumane care for patients. Once we shift from rhetoric to action, however, it seems that we cannot say unambiguously that quality-of-life considerations play or must play a central role in clinical decisions, even to give an adequate account of much of current practice, especially with adult patients. Furthermore, it is certainly not true that humane care requires any such premise. Admittedly, the amount of data on actual decision-making practices is not very large and several quite substantial lacunae exist in what is available. Yet I think that whatever data exist do not demonstrate a need for quality-of-life concerns in this process. I draw this conclusion from three sources: my own experience, available studies of physician decision making, and reviews of published guidelines for "do not resuscitate" orders.

The experience of the author in critical cases

The first of these is my own experience in teaching and observation in a clinical setting. From 1978–83 I was a member of the clinical medical-ethics faculty at the University of Tennes-

235

see Center for the Health Sciences. During most of that time, I coordinated a monthly series in which cases were presented and the moral issues discussed with clinicians, medical students, and residents. Over a four-year period, at least a dozen cases dealt with the same issues—life and death, treatment or nontreatment—that concern us here. Of these cases, and the much larger number encountered in the hospital itself, only a very few clearly seemed to require the quality-of-life judgments that are so prominent in the rhetoric of the contemporary discussion. The vast majority of cases concerned patients with either a known terminal disease, such as advanced cancer of the colon, or a combination of medical problems such that one could not say that further attempts at aggressive therapy would probably save the life of the patient. A case that illustrates this point especially well is that of Mr. R.

> Mr. R was a forty-three year old white male originally in satisfactory health but with a known bicuspid aortic valve for two years. He was admitted to a local hospital with fever and confusion. Cardiac evaluation revealed a new aortic insufficiency and blood cultures showed a staph infection with evidence of multiple emboli to the brain, left knee, and right foot. The patient was started on Nafcillin for subacute bacterial endocarditis. Later the patient developed congestive heart failure and an aortic prosthesis was inserted. During recovery from surgery the patient developed a cereberal hemorrage in the right occipital area. The clot was removed but the patient was compromised by a left hemiparesis and global aphasia, with particularly notable receptive deficits. The patient's fever returned and further evaluation showed a return of staph aureus. The patient's aortic insufficiency also returned and another prosthesis was judged to be necessary. However the patient was also judged to be a very poor risk for surgery and no procedure was done. A gallium scan showed a lesion in the left kidney that was found to be renal cell carcinoma. The kidney was removed with no gross evidence of metastasis.

At this point the patient remained a wasted white male who looked much older than his age and required total care. He was unresponsive to verbal stimuli, but he could vocalize recognizable English words in an inconsistent pattern. Without a new aortic prosthesis, the patient could not be sustained indefinitely. His wife, however, insisted that everything possible be done for him. She would not consider stopping his antibiotics and she demanded that surgery be done. She was constantly at his bedside holding his hand and watching him. Since his eyes were open, she believed that he was often looking at her. He also occasionally spoke English words in a voice she knew and loved. From these factors she felt that he would recover and return to his former life.

Mr. R. was dying. Without surgery his cardiac insufficiency was certain to cause his death; in his extremely debilitated condition, he was a poor candidate for surgery: very likely, he would not survive it. Thus it seems clear that neither we nor the physicians needed to resort to quality-of-life considerations to conclude that further aggressive therapy, and even further use of the respirator, was not humane care for Mr. R.[2] We shall return to the nuances of this case below.[3] For now I simply note that this case was far more representative of those we found in our grand-rounds series than ones in which quality-of-life considerations necessarily dominated the discussion.

Studies of physician decision making

This conclusion is not, I believe, disproven by the available studies of physician decision making in similar cases, particularly of adult, incompetent patients. The most important of these studies is that by Diana Crane.[4] Professor Crane acknowledges that her studies do not show a straightforward concern for quality-of-life considerations in clinical decisions. Rather, two conclusions emerge: 1) physicians vary greatly in willingness to use aggressive means to save life, and 2) physicians apparently esteem normal mental function significantly more than physical integrity in decision making. Many more physicians would use aggressive treatment with patients who would remain physically disabled than would in the cases of patients who remain mentally disabled after therapy. She concludes that many physicians place a higher value on social interaction than on mere bodily life; as a result, they are more willing to let patients die for this "quality of life" reason.[5]

Professor Crane's data will bear out her conclusion only if the cases that physicians are asked to reflect upon can be clearly classed as quality-of-life cases, not as cases in which the prognosis is poor or doubtful. Moreover, only if such quality-of-life factors would be essential to achieve what would be widely regarded as a proper outcome, will this data affect my argument. For these purposes she groups her cases into four sets, on the basis of two pairs of terms: those where the patient is salvageable and those where he is not; and those involving either physical or mental disability.[6] But this key word *salvageable* is ambiguous. For example, it could be claimed that Mr. R. is a salvageable patient. His life might be prolonged with surgery. Given his very wasted condition and his cancer, however, it is unlikely that his life can be saved indefinitely, whatever is done at this point. Thus, seen from a limited point of view one might classify this patient as salvageable and view a decision to withhold treatment as necessarily involving quality-of-life factors. Seen from a broader perspective, however, that is surely not the only manner in which this case might be seen.

It appears on inspection that Professor Crane presents some cases, particularly of adult patients, with similar ambiguity. In some cases information is presented that may very well be crucial in making the decision but which is not strictly of a medical or quality-of-life sort: such as whether a family is pressing for aggressive care or is willing to care for a stroke victim.[7] Particularly when the family either presses for aggressive care or is unwilling to sanction it, the physician might feel that he or she will face legal difficulties if he or she does not proceed as the family wishes. In other cases the information as presented does not draw out the quality-of-life factor as strikingly as would be necessary to reach the conclusions that quality-of-life advocates may wish to reach.

Consider, for example, the cases presented to neurosurgeons in which patients with intracerebral hematoma were considered. In one case the hematoma is described as "large, left, deep frontal," while in the second it is described as being in the "nondominant right parietal-occipital" area. In the first case, the patient would have residual mental impairment; in the second, visual field restriction and left hemiparesis. Yet the first case states that "although transcortical incision with direct surgical evacuation of the hematoma might prove fatal, he might also die if the hematoma is not evacuated."[8] This surely adds another and perhaps important piece of information that could be crucial in deciding on surgery. In the second case the reader is simply told that the patient may die without surgery. These are subtle but important differences in the way the cases are presented. These differences may very well be decisive in determining whether one operates on a patient or not. Yet these differences do not center on quality-of-life considerations.

Aside from the cases in which the patient is dying or the success of treatment is doubtful, another group of her cases presents situations in which a terminal diagnosis is suspected but not confirmed, or where an acute problem is superimposed on one of longer duration. In the former category is a case where the patient has a lung mass which the radiologist suspects is cancer and the patient becomes severely dyspneic before a biopsy can be done. In the latter category is a case where a patient has had a lung removed as a result of cancer and then suffers a heart attack. These cases could be resolved in many different ways. But even a resolution that concludes that treatment ought to be withheld, could be reached on grounds independent of belief that any of these patients have or will have a "life not worth living" even after treatment.[9]

These problems are even noted in the questions that are asked of pediatricians and pediatric surgeons concerning the treatment of severely abnormal newborns. Sometimes the crucial distinction is whether the parents are said to want the child or are pressing for treatment. For example, in one version of a case involving an infant with Down's syndrome, the mother is described as being thirty-five with a history of miscarriage and wanting the child very much while another version says just the reverse insofar as the wishes of the family are concerned. Such complicating details obscure the question of whether quality-of-life considerations need play or have played a crucial role in reaching a just resolution to these cases or explain the results obtained by Professor Crane.[10]

It is true that some of Professor Crane's cases and the data she obtains are best interpreted in quality-of-life terms. In other words, they are best interpreted by viewing the choice made by the physician as one involving the degree of mental impairment that the patient would live with even after treatment. However, not all of these cases can unambiguously be so interpreted; therefore, it seems to me that her data do not as strongly imply as it may seem the necessary role of these factors in such a substantial amount of practice as to make my policy unwise or unworkable.

Close analysis of other recent studies seem to support this general conclusion, although they may be thought to provide evidence of the central importance of quality-of-life factors in clinical decision making. In one recent study, the case presented to physicians for a decision described a patient with an acute exacerbation of chronic obstructive pulmonary disease. At the time of the decision, he needed to be placed on a respirator. But the condition of this patient was such that it is difficult to say that his life could be saved or sustained indefinitely, even with aggressive therapy. In other words, it does not present a case in which quality-of-life considerations will necessarily be decisive in determining clinical action. Both prognostic and quality-of-life projection might ground a decision non to treat; it would be impossible to tell from the data as presented which of these factors predominated in any particular physician's decision.[11]

Further, in a recent review of actual decisions not to treat fever in nursing homes, prognosis played a crucial role in non-treatment decisions, as did other factors that may also be closely related to prognosis, such as deterioration in the general functioning of the patient. In fact this factor of general patient deterioration was the best single predictor of a nontreatment decision. Deterioration, however, can mean either a slipping from one level of mental or physiological functioning or a slipping from living to dying by the patient. Especially for patients with multiple problems, such as those in nursing homes, it will often be difficult to separate these meanings with precision.

This fact itself renders any conclusion about the centrality of quality-of-life factors doubtful.[12]

These observations seem to be borne out also by the literature describing nontreatment decisions, even in infant cases. To be sure there is a body of opinion and practice that deliberately withholds treatment on quality-of-life grounds. To this we shall return later. What appears in some reports of actual decisions is, however, the fact that a very substantial proportion of those newborns that are not treated are those who have such major abnormalities that treatment either definitely cannot or may not be able to save their lives. In Duff and Campbell's classic paper, which started much of the current debate on these practices, 86 per cent of the deaths in their newborn center over a two and a half year period involved infants with specific pathologic conditions.[13] The remaining cases involved a conscious decision to withhold treatment that might have sustained life. But even here their description of some of their actual cases suggests that many of these infants had a doubtful prognosis, even with appropriate therapy. Consider this one case that they report:

> Another child had chronic pulmonary disease after positive pressure ventilation with high oxygen concentrations for treatment of severe idiopathic respiratory distress syndrome. By five months of age he still required forty per cent oxygen to survive and even then he was chronically dyspneic and cyanotic. He also suffered from *cor pulmonale* which was difficult to control with digoxin and diuretics.[14]

Even under the best of circumstances, this child has a poor prognosis. His respiratory function is weak and he cannot be maintained indefinitely on supplemental oxygen. It seems, therefore, that we need not describe this case in any way that involves a quality-of-life determination. It is sufficient to say that his prognosis is poor to reach the outcome that these authors reached: further attempts at therapy should be withheld.

In another paper, Duff himself describes another case in which the selective nontreatment of a newborn on quality-of-life grounds is supposedly justified.

241

Baby girl U illustrates these problems. Apparently in good health at birth, she developed symptoms of bowel obstruction (from a malformation) at thirty-four hours of age. At surgery, most of her necrotic bowel was removed to save her life. Intravenous nutrition was given in hope of eventual adequate bowel function. However, such substitutions commonly have complications as happened in this case, and they cannot be effective in the long run. By four months of age, intravenous support was increasingly problematic and the bowel was not functioning. While the baby received every advantage of treatment, she had been put through several operations and had endured constant manipulations and treatments.[15]

As Duff himself notes, this infant had a very poor prognosis from the moment that the surgery removed such a large portion of the bowel. To justify any decision to withhold further aggressive care for this infant, we would not need any recourse to quality-of-life factors such as distress or suffering. We need only focus on the very fact that Duff himself notes: namely, that this child has "perhaps less than one chance in ten thousand" of long-term survival.

It is true that these authors and others advocate nontreatment for a much broader range of cases on fairly clear quality-of-life grounds, such as withholding surgery from Down's syndrome infants with intestinal atresia; yet I submit that their own classic paper as well as other reports in the literature show that much practice, even for newborns, can be accounted for without recourse to the necessary use of quality-of-life factors, which are often mistakenly thought to be crucial in these very cases. In the most recent and important study in this area, the vast preponderance of cases from an intensive care unit where do not resuscitate orders were written involved patients with a very grim prognosis. Only 24 per cent of the cases mentioned quality-of-life factors; even some of these also mentioned either a grim prognosis or the wishes of the patient.[16]

Aside from this slender body of empirical data, we can look at established hospital guidelines on the use of "no code" orders for evidence on what is viewed as acceptable contemporary practice in withholding such life-saving medical care. An examination of those guidelines that have appeared in print, however, supports the conclusions I have drawn from my own experience and from a review of published data.[17]

Guidelines on "Do Not Resuscitate" Orders

For example, a medical-legal committee of the bar and medical associations in San Francisco writes that "DNR—do not resuscitate—orders are appropriately recommended when the patient suffers from a known lethal disease" which cannot be cured.[18] This same view, limiting the DNR order to terminally ill patients, appears in other published hospital guidelines, such as those prepared for the hospitals operated by Los Angeles County and the University of Wisconsin Hospital.[19] Many other published guidelines do not specify the grounds for issuing a DNR order. Never are quality-of-life factors indicated as an acceptable foundation, by themselves, for physician or family decision making in these cases.

It therefore appears that on the basis of the available evidence, contemporary medical practice is not so inseparably wedded to quality-of-life considerations as to render the policy developed here impotent or inhumane. In all studies a very sizeable percentage of physicians would pursue aggressive therapy even in cases where the patient's life could very probably not be sustained indefinitely. In some other instances, the cases themselves do not unambiguously show that quality-of-life factors must predominate in decision making. Most important, none of these studies show that even what passes for quality-of-life judgments in these terms are necessary parts of humane and compassionate care.

Feasibility of the New Policy

Since contemporary practice does not seem to exclude the policy I have articulated in earlier chapters, we may ask whether it should. Will this exclusion of quality-of-life factors lead to patently inhumane and unjust forms of medical care? To ask this question is to ask just how policy would affect practice. How would it affect physicians and patients?

All reflection on practical choice, in any human endeavor, begins with a description of that which is to be done. This description is itself not morally neutral.[20] In cases of actual choice we do not bifurcate our lives in such a fact/value manner. Unless my actions have some value to me, I can scarcely be called a human agent at all. Human action is a conscious pursuit of some end that is seen as worthwhile. If my bodily movements are to be viewed as human actions and not the wild thrashing of inchoate forces or animalistic drives, they must be seen as a product of such an evaluative choice. Thus the meaning of an action will be disclosed in the first instance by the terms of reference within which I am led to see it and evaluate it.

For example, suppose I give ten dollars to a very wealthy person. If this act is described simply as one of generosity on my part, it would seem that if another person could benefit more from such generosity, I ought to give him or her this money: say, if my child would derive more pleasure from a new toy than a rich man from a pittance he does not need, then the correct course of action seem clear—buy the toy. But if my act is described as repaying a debt, then the evaluation seems to change. In such a case it seems doubtful that I could simply throw my money around as if the fact of my debt did not matter. It would seem that if I am to spend my money otherwise than to pay the debt, my reasons must be more serious and of a different sort than the mere happiness or pleasure of others.

These are elementary considerations, given some voice in a wide variety of moral philosophies. Yet they do make us aware that the context in which an action is viewed is of central significance in evaluating and choosing. One way of seeing the act closes off some choices as unacceptable: I may not neglect a debt to buy dinner for a friend. It can also lead to a presumption, perhaps refutable, that a certain course of action is required. But it does not answer all the questions that can properly be raised about individual cases of choice and action. In this manner, I submit, the policy conclusions arrived at earlier function best as a gestalt that orders the field of our vision before choice. In this manner, they supply us with a framework within which we can seek humane resolutions to the most difficult choices that now press on us in medicine. This framework allows us to act in one way when we can reasonably describe a case as one of mercifully ceasing therapy that cannot or may not save the patient from his or her terminal course, and prohibits us from acting in other ways when one can be saved. It allows us to act with mercy but prohibits the taking of life sometimes done under its banner.

If I am right, the proper context for an acceptable decision in the most difficult of these cases will be a search for the kind of care that can save a patient's life over a long time. In the vast majority of cases, this inquiry will generate an obvious conclusion: a patient with an acute infectious process, such as pneumonia, needs life-saving antibiotics which will eliminate the disease and return him or her to health. Such a patient stands at one end of a spectrum—nontreatment is unacceptable. At the other end of this spectrum are those cases in which further therapy is either optional or wrong. Such may be the case with a patient with end-stage liver disease or with a cancer that is inoperable and untreatable, such as cancer of the pancreas.

While many actual cases may fit into one of these two groupings, the distinction itself is by no means as sharp as some would like it to be; some cases will fall in an area of uncertainty between these two poles.[21] This gray area appears in two ways. First are those cases where prognosis is doubtful or uncertain, such as where the relevant data shows only a 30–40 per cent chance of five-year survival with treatment. Second are those cases of chronic illness that may be fatal but not for some years: for example, progressive degenerative diseases—whether vascular, such as Beurger's Disease or neuromuscular, such as Lou Gehrig's disease—are fatal but not for some years. Some cases from my own experience I think highlight many of these gray areas of uncertain prognosis and difficult judgment.

> Mr. C is a sixty-five-year-old man with a history of hypertension, diabetes, and stroke. He had become progressively confused and disoriented over the past few months after

245

a lengthy hospital stay for treatment of recurrent gastric ulceration which resulted in a partial gastrectomy. He had been experiencing severe diarrhea, weakness, and lethargy since his operation and subsequently became debilitated to the point of being unable to care for himself, restricted to his bed with frequent episodes of delirium. On the day of admission, the patient had an acute onset of complete unresponsiveness, with eyes fixed to the left followed by vomiting and decerebrate posturing. On arriving in the emergency room, the patient was hypotensive and exhibited neurological findings suggestive of a right MCA-CVA— a stroke in the right side of the brain—with several other metabolic problems, and a urinary tract infection. He was initially treated with aggressive fluid therapy, sodium bicarbonate, and antibiotics. The patient remained unresponsive to all stimuli except deep pain. On the third hospital day, he experienced twelve hours of anuria, followed by insertion of a CVP line and treatment with fluids and a diuretic. Several hours later the patient developed a consolidation in the lower left lung, which was followed with an expansion of his antibiotic coverage. He remained in a stable but critical condition for the next week and experienced multiple problems with fluid and electrolyte imbalances. A Dobbhoff tube was inserted for continuous feedings and he began passing large amounts of watery stool, which were caused by his rapid processing of food intake due to the removal of part of his stomach. This required daily changes in his nutritional and electrolyte intake. His neurological status did improve to the point where he was conscious and could squeeze the hand of a person talking to him. He remained verbally uncommunicative and at this point a nursing home placement was being sought.

Mr. C is clearly in a serious condition. It would appear that he cannot survive indefinitely in his condition, especially because of his need for continued electrolyte replacement, which is difficult if not impossible to maintain successfully. At the same time, however, we cannot predict when this patient will die or what will cause his death. Several of his medical problems could be fatal; whether they will is only partially under human control. At this point with continued aggressive therapy we may stand some chance of salvaging his life and sending him to a nursing home for a short while; but this prognosis is uncertain at best.

Note, however, the difference between this sort of discussion—revolving around the prognosis of a difficult case—and a discussion of whether this patient has a "low quality-of-life," and thus must be brought to death either actively or passively. To analyse the case in terms of low quality-of-life leads directly to the conceptual and practical morass noted in the earlier chapters of this book.[22] We would need to know what such a quality-of-life is, what constitutes its absence and how much of its presence is necessary for the patient to be "worth saving." In these cases we are not merely uncertain about the application of a rule to the case; we do not even know what the rule should be. Moreover, an attempt to resolve this case in quality-of-life terms would entail that at some point we would conclude that this life is not worth saving, not that its prognosis is grim or doubtful. In other words, a decision along such lines will include the most troubling judgment of all, that some human beings are excluded from the moral compact that protects the equal worth of us all.

This point is fundamental. There is a crucial difference between these two sources of uncertainty regarding the force of a rule in a given case, one of which is fatal to the rule itself. In the first case, the rule itself is defective for we cannot tell what its range of application is to be; in the second, the rule is clear, though we may have difficulty with locating a complex case in regard to it.

Take any rule that prohibits an act: the complete statement of the rule, with exceptions, will be RE. In any situation of choice, we need to know whether a given act is covered by RE or not. If the rule is acceptable, it will state clearly the range of its application and the nature of its exceptions. But all rules, especially rules of law and policy, have a measure of what Hart terms "open texture": that is, the rulemaker cannot possibly foresee every set of future circumstances and every conflict of rules; thus any given rule cannot possibly state precisely how it ought to apply in every future case.[23] For example, a well-established common law rule forbids parents from depriving their children of necessary medical care. Such a rule obviously conflicts with another rule that allows parents to raise their children as they see fit. In the context of specific religious tenets that may forbid certain types of care, in conjoining these two rules, a class of exceptions was created in cases in which medical care may be desirable but is not necessary to save the life of the child. Hence the rule with exceptions has come to be that life-saving medical care must be provided to the child; otherwise the wishes of the parent will be respected.

In the vast majority of cases, this rule is clear enough to generate reasonable solutions and specify punishable lapses. Sometimes, however, we simply do not know whether to say that the therapy is necessary life-saving care, like the removal of a ruptured appendix, or an experimental treatment with perhaps only a small hope of saving the child's life. The rule itself remains clear, however, as does the exception. If the case can be viewed as unnecessary treatment, the child need not be subjected to it. But if it is necessary, and likely to save his or her life, it must be provided. Once the case can be located with respect to the rule, the resolution follows.

In other cases, a rule itself may violate one of the core aspects of what Fuller calls the "internal morality of law," for when a law is so unclear as to leave its object unspecified, it fails as law.[24] The rule may be stated in such a fashion as to invite confusion or absurdity. This point does not commit us to any view regarding the substance of the rule itself; a given rule may be plausible as a rule and still permit what we would believe to be very great injustice. For example, a rule that permitted a person to kill anyone who trespasses on his or her property would seem to be wildly unacceptable. Yet it does clearly specify its object and cannot be attacked on this ground. On the other hand, an exception clause that permits one to murder another whenever one subjectively believes that one's honor has been challenged simply cannot be viewed as part of an adequate rule. The exception clause is so expansive that almost any instance of murder can be excepted; the exception is so vague as to evacuate the applicability of the rule itself.

248

These observations are crucial in helping us answer the claim that the policy outlined above can no more give clear answers in specific cases than a quality-of-life policy. In one sense this is a trivial truism: all rules regarding complex areas of human life that are imperfectly foreseen and grasped in language have some open texture. But the objection that trades on this truism simply misses the point. The earlier chapters amply demonstrated that a quality-of-life policy provides us no idea what the complete rule should be. In this respect any such policy is bound to join both sources of rule uncertainty noted above. As such, it will necessarily create a far greater range of uncertainty in specific cases than does mine. Again, in cases of unclarity or conflict between rules, the quality-of-life proposals ask us to appeal to higher order principles that plainly contradict the most fundamental constitutive principles of our communal life, principles that lie behind the specific rules against murder or child neglect themselves.[25]

In this respect the use of a quality-of-life framework for decision making is bound to swallow up all other principles, just as philosophers have noticed that the use of " beneficence" principles has in moral theory. In cases of conflict we are forced to resort to the higher order principle that permits a resolution among specific rules. In the cases we are considering, a quality-of-life framework entails not only vagueness in the application of rule to cases and patent disparities in the results achieved; it finally results in a fundamental departure from what our polity has historically accepted as its most central principle.

Such a judgment follows only if we view cases like that of Mr. C in terms of a "quality-of-life" gestalt. A humane resolution to the problems of this case, however, does not require us to frame the case in these terms. It could just as plausibly be concluded that Mr. C cannot be kept alive on this basis indefinitely and that, as a result, further therapy may be withheld on these grounds.

Mr. C's case falls in this gray area of uncertain prognosis. In other cases this uncertainty appears as a looming backdrop over an otherwise unproblematic situation. Consider the case of Ricky:

Ricky is a five-year-old boy with chronic renal disease. He has had six operations for this problem already. At this point the renal condition is judged stable but it is uncertain how long this will last. He could go into renal failure immediately or his stable condition could last several years. The attending nephrologist cannot be sure, though he suggests that a stable prognosis for at least a year is more likely. A year ago the parents were approached concerning a transplant and they refused. They had already been through five operations with Ricky and they were reluctant to consider further procedures, especially something as major as a transplant. They felt that Ricky had been through enough and that it would be best—if he had to die—that he do so sooner. They had two other children, seven and three, and the strain on their emotions and family finances was beginning to be serious. The older sister especially resented the parents' heavy involvement with Ricky. Six months ago Ricky developed seizures, following a sixth, relatively simple surgical procedure on his one functioning kidney. After the procedure his condition stabilized as noted above, but his seizures continued. He was seen by a neurologist but the parent refused to allow him to perform a complete workup to determine the etiology of the seizures. They did permit pharmacological treatment of the seizures themselves. The treatment was only partially effective. After several months the neurologist strongly recommended that the child be hospitalized, at least to allow a systematic attempt to control the seizures. His parents reluctantly permitted this. On admission the child was treated with several different seizure medications with only moderate success. At one point the child was having a prolonged *grand mal* seizure which was unresponsive to normal medication. At this point the neurologist began administration of very high doses of phenobarbitol to control the seizures. One possible effect of such doses is respiratory arrest. When the patient began experiencing dyspnea, the neurologist ordered the use of a respirator to avoid the possibility of total arrest. The parents refused, stating that the child had suffered enough.

250

Like Mr. C's, Ricky's long term prognosis was uncertain. If his kidneys failed again, it was doubtful that they could be repaired surgically, and—at his age and condition—chronic dialysis was not likely to succeed. Therefore it might be concluded that further aggressive therapy would have no real benefit for him, and may be forsaken.

But this conclusion holds only for his renal condition. It may be justified to withhold therapy if his kidneys failed again. His seizures are another matter. At this point we do not have enough information to make any judgment about the seizures, their etiology, prognosis, and complications. We cannot even say that the prognosis is uncertain. On inspection it may turn out to be a simple matter of getting the right dosage and mix of drugs. Until we can get more information, we must treat the seizures as aggressively as his parents will permit. Moreover, even if the prognosis were doubtful about the seizures themselves, it would not follow that we should acquiesce in the parental request not to use the respirator. Ricky's respiratory problem is iatrogenic, that is, it is due to his therapy. Only because the amount of medication he is receiving depresses his respiratory functioning does he have this problem. Since we do not know the etiology of his seizures or the medication that will be necessary to control them, it seems that we must treat these reversible side effects, at least until we are more certain of the etiology and prognosis of the seizures.

All these uncertainties of our judgment, however, prescind from the framework within which this case is viewed, one that focuses our attention on the possible life-saving benefit further treatment may offer Ricky. Again, here it appears that a focus which attached importance to the quality-of-life of the patient or his family would easily generate a different conclusion, even to the point of overlooking the iatrogenic nature of his respiratory distress. The family is obviously under stress from Ricky's medical problems; Ricky himself certainly is undergoing some distress and perhaps suffering from his condition. A decision-making framework that focused our attention on such "quality-

of-life" indicators might surely find it easy to justify withholding treatment, although Ricky is not dying; indeed, at present it
is not even known that his prognosis is uncertain.

In these two cases the future is uncertain and no decision-
making framework can make it less so. The judgment about
what is to be done in each case will reflect these uncertainties.
What the judgment need not reflect or imply is a belief that
either of these patients have lives that do not merit the most
primitive of our civic rights.

These uncertainties are even more pronounced in cases
where the prognosis is that the patient is terminally ill, but
where his or her death will not come for several years. Consider
in this regard the case of Mr. P:

> Mr. P was a fifty-one-year-old white male who presented to
> the clinic with a chief complaint of weakness and muscle
> tremors, especially in his hands. He was in apparent good
> health until approximately six months ago, when he
> started noticing that he could not do all of the physical
> activity he normally did. On further examination he was
> found to have the beginnings of spasticity in his legs, exag-
> gerated deep reflexes, and a pronounced Babinski reflex.
> Combined with pathological data, a positive diagnosis of
> Lou Gehrig's disease—amyotrophic lateral sclerosis—was
> made. It was estimated that the disease was in its early
> stages and that while it was almost certainly fatal, the pa-
> tient could expect two or three more years of life. Further-
> more, while the increasing lack of neuromuscular capacity
> would require more physical care, at no time would he
> suffer deficits in his mental capacity. When told of his situa-
> tion, Mr. P initially became depressed, but with supportive
> psychotherapy he resolved to continue as much of his pre-
> vious life as possible. Since he was a computer expert, his
> employment was not jeopardized.
>
> Nine months later Mr. P was seen for follow-up, at
> which time he complained of worsening shortness of
> breath. He was admitted for a workup which revealed no
> cause for his respiratory distress, except for his disease,
> which usually involved these sequelae. Upon learning that
> he would need to spend the rest of his life on a respirator,

he refused. He stated that he did not want to live for two years "attached to this damn machine." If he could not survive "on my own, in my own house," then "let me die now."

Mr. P was dying. His disease was progressive and fatal. But his terminal course was likely to be prolonged and the time he would spend attached to a respirator would also be prolonged. Whether it would be right to withhold the respirator at this point would be a difficult matter to judge. Mr. P surely can do many things and can undertake significant activities during his illness. But the respirator cannot in any manner save his life; it can only delay the inevitable course of his disease. Thus at least here, the respirator can be viewed as an appendage that cannot save the patient's life and can, therefore, be forsaken on these grounds.

At this point it is instructive to note the difference in the cases of Mr. P and Mr. A, who was encountered in our discussion of suicide.[26] Mr. A had a degenerative disease of the vascular system. In his case a depressive illness was superimposed on the primary vascular problem, a depression almost certainly caused by the slow, inevitable course of his disease. But Mr. A's depression was treatable, and had responded to treatment in the past. Furthermore, Mr. A did not require our assistance in killing himself; he was a very intelligent man—if he ever decided to kill himself, he would not show up at the hospital seeking help. Therefore, irrespective of what we might conclude about his right to kill himself, he did not need the assistance of anyone in carrying out such a plan. No public policy need be framed to deal with such a case.

Furthermore, Mr. A was clearly suffering from a major depressive episode, one that was diagnosed on the basis of several clinical indicators other than his statement concerning suicide. Given his depressed state and his obvious ambivalence about suicide, Mr. A did not present in an unambiguous fashion the question of the right of a clearly competent patient to opt for death over life. Mr. P, however, has none of these impediments to his competency. As such his case represents in the clearest possible terms the question of his right to opt for death and our role in helping him do so.

It seems intuitively obvious that Mr. P retains the liberty to choose for himself whether to forgo further therapy, although he can use this liberty foolishly. This liberty would seem to still be present even if he had an acute disease for which he refused obviously life-saving care, such as refusing antibiotics for pneumonia or blood transfusions or routine surgery. As we noted above, cases in this latter category are difficult to distinguish from suicide.[27] As such, it is likewise very problematic to assert that the patient has a natural or human right to so act in a morally dubious way. At the very least, the justification of any such natural or human right would have to proceed in a manner fundamentally different from the justification of most other specific rights.[28] In the typical case we say that person has a "right to do X"—such as to bear or to beget a child. In making this claim we single out from among the enormous diversity of human activities a specific act and we assert that only very serious and stringently defined reasons will justify interference with this specific activity. But this special moral status cannot possibly pertain to every act that the individual may wish to perform. What we obviously do is select out of all human endeavors those that we regard with special significance. These the individual is said to have a "right" to do.

This point is recognized even by strong rights theorists such as Childress and Dworkin, who disavow the notion of a broad liberty right if that is described as a licence to do as one pleases. Liberty as licence is far too broad, as Dworkin notes, to stand by itself as a fundamental right. But Dworkin's focus on liberty as independence is unhelpful here. For him liberty as independence arranges the various liberties of the person in a hierarchy. But this need to rank actions and states of being according to some standard of moral or nonmoral importance only proves the point just made. Secondly, any right to "equal respect" or to respect for one's "life plans" simply does not reach the questions raised in practice. What we want to know is which personal actions and choices are to be covered by the principle of respect for personal integrity and which are not. If a curfew is equivalent to a forced sterilization program as an assault on liberty as independence, then we are back with the untenable liberty as licence. But if this is true, then the distinction among human acts required to transcend liberty as licence cannot based on the subjective importance of the act to the individual. It must require some concept of the proper life for man and the forms of activity conducive to and part of that life.[29] This significance is itself patently moral. In other words the class of activities that we say an individual has a right to pursue only comes into view in light of a more comprehensive and more communal vision of the moral life itself. For example, to say that a person has a right to do something such as practice a religion of one's own choosing is to say that this activity is an integral part of the moral life. Therefore it can be overridden only for the most serious reasons, since in overriding one's right, we affect one's capacity for the moral life, not just his or her private desires or concerns. On the other hand, walking the streets late at night or driving a car at a certain speed may not be nearly as coeval with the moral life as religious worship; as such, a curfew or a speed limit may be imposed for reasons of public order or safety far more easily than any restrictions on child bearing or the freedom to worship.

This connection between moral rights and the morally right and good *per se* lies at the center of the doctrine of human rights that is much discussed in contemporary literature. Without it most of our conventional beliefs about human or moral rights are plainly incoherent. Grant it, however, and you grant implicitly that the right to engage in actions that are morally wrong or dubious will have to be justified in ways that differ fundamentally from the justification of acts that are widely held to be right or good in themselves. In the liberal theory of rights, a crucial distinction is between rights justified as part of the moral life and rights justified as a matter of prudence either because we are skeptical about our own moral knowledge or because the apparatus necessary for intervention is onerous, dangerous or cumbersome.[30]

In the cases we are considering, involving completely competent patients who would undertake a course of action that almost certainly will lead to their death, these observations are important. When such a patient removes himself or herself from therapy, it cannot be plausibly concluded that one's action is moral correct nor need it be for us to avoid an onerous imposition on personal liberty. We noted in an earlier chapter that these cases involve the tension between liberty and equal worth in the most direct manner possible.[31] To allow the patient to pursue one's path in these matters does not require us either to accept one's assessment of the situation at hand or to agree that one has a fundamental right to die that is at stake. To respect the patient's choice, we need only to conclude that a policy that permitted intervention over the objections of the person would entail such onerous acts in practice and would set such a paternalistic example for other cases that it is unwise and unworkable. In these cases liberty follows from prudence.[32]

In such a manner liberty is preserved in a practical manner for what are eminently practical reasons. But often the choice between liberty and equality is not posed in such a direct and compelling manner, either because the competency of the patient to choose one's own care is compromised or because one either does not come for treatment or cannot be treated effectively. In any of these situations, the direct tension between liberty and equal worth is not presented and no choice between these goods need be made.

For clearly competent patients who refuse plainly life-saving therapy, such a choice is presented in the clearest possible terms. But here the respect for the autonomous choice of the patient that must be granted on practical grounds does not entail any conclusion about the quality of life of the patient and does not require us to agree with one's choice. Viewed as such, the patient's choice does not pose a challenge to the horizon within which policy must be framed in our sort of regime. Three aspects of contemporary practice, however, do appear, at this writing to be at odds with the conclusions I have reached:

1. abortion on demand,
2. care for certain types of seriously abnormal newborns,
3. the care of permanently comatose patients.

These differences will only be of importance insofar as the horizon within which I believe choice must be made will lead to serious harms or wrongs in any of these instances. If such is not likely to happen, then the fact of contemporary practice is irrelevant to my conclusions.

Abortion we may dismiss briefly, The aborting woman wants an otherwise normal human being not to exist merely because she believes that it will be better for her if this death is brought about. Once the human standing of the fetus is admitted, however, I do not see how contemporary practices in this regard can be sustained in any reasonable terms that preserve even a semblance of the notion of equal worth. In this sense contemporary abortion practice is so at odds with the most primitive of our civic commitments that it seems impossible to sustain it. That this rejection of contemporary practice would inconvenience some people I readily admit. But to allay inconvenience at the price of the death of other human beings is so incommensurate and so much a departure from our tradition that it is difficult to conceive of any serious basis for contemporary practice.[33] The one conceivable exception to this conclusion may be thought to be the case of a fetus that is genetically or developmentally abnormal. In such cases it may be supposed that the harm of continued existence is so great to that individual human being that it creates serious difficulties for any policy prohibiting abortion in such cases. In theory these cases are indistinguishable from selective infanticide and all of the difficulties noted earlier in these cases will obtain here. This follows for two reasons. First, selective abortion on these grounds cannot be done before receiving test results demonstrating deformity, and abortion on these grounds cannot be done before about nineteen–twenty weeks gestational age.[34] By this time the fetus has virtually complete morphological development and can only be described as a human being, indistinguishable from the neonate. Furthermore, the very rationale of these abortions is indistinguishable from that offered for infanticide: death is preferable to life in a deformed state.

At this point, however, contemporary practice in selective abortion or infanticide is almost impossible to sustain. As we have seen earlier,[35] the case made for contemporary practice is so vaguely worded that it cannot offer much guidance for practice in sorting out which types of medical care in which types of cases may be withdrawn. This follows because the key concepts that supposedly specify an acceptable quality of life are impossible to define fairly. From the viewpoint of practice, however, we should note that often where death is actually sought, especially in selective abortion, any claim that life is worse then death looks patently absurd. This is especially true about selective abortion. Here the two most common cases are a fetus with Down's syndrome or with a neural tube defect (NTD), that is, spina bifida. But where is the widely recognizable harm in Down's syndrome? Most such children are retarded but the vast majority are not profoundly retarded nor are they physically handicapped or faced with lives of pain or suffering. They learn to walk and talk and enjoy simple pleasures in life. Not knowing the lives they cannot lead, they do not suffer much from such knowledge.[36] In the light of these facts, the contemporary practice of preferring death over life to fetuses faced with such lives rapidly seems absurd. It is even more so when one considers the impossibility of knowing much more about the fetus or neonate than that he or she has the disorder, trisomy 21. *In utero* that is all we can know. We cannot know anything about other morphological abnormalities nor about how the person will respond to his or her difficulties, how he or she will feel about life. Any supposition about the quality of such a life will be sheer guesswork and a policy based on it is difficult to sustain.

These same absurdities are seen in the cases of fetuses or infants with a NTD. *In utero* about all we can determine is that the fetus has an open lesion in the spinal column.[37] But this fact tells us little that is useful for practice, since more than 60% of such children will have normal intelligence, a fact that must be crucial in any quality-of-life judgment. *Ex utero* the situation changes little. Even in the worst prognostic category, a majority of the children will have IQs in the normal range following aggressive therapy.[38] They will not, as a rule, lead lives filled with pain and sorrow. Suffering on the other hand arises from one's relation to one's environment—a thing impossible to know at this stage of one's life.

In general, then, contemporary practice of selective abortion or infanticide cannot be sustained, even on its own quality-of-life terms; there is no evidence that changing practice would increase individual misery or harm. Even abstracting from the definitional problems associated with such a standard, clearly to opt for death on these grounds we would need to choose death for many children who would not necessarily have lives of pain and suffering and sorrow. Even the utilitarian morality to which many practicioners seem attached would not justify such a choice.

This conclusion does not deny that some infants will have multiple abnormalities or serious problems that render their prognosis uncertain, even with the best of care; there will always be the "Baby Janes" of the world and a discerning judgment will always be required in such cases. But this conclusion does not apply to the vast majority of cases in which selective abortion occurs.

Of all the cases confronted in practice, the most perplexing for the position I have taken are those of patients in permanent coma or what is termed in clinical jargon a "persistent vegetative state," such as Karen Quinlan.

Miss Quinlan was not dead, and—in the usual sense—she could not be described as dying. But neither was she in pain or suffering. Removing her from the respirator could not therefore be justified in any of the normal quality-of-life ways. Yet the nearly universal judgment of serious opinion was that removal of the respirator was the right thing to do.[39] It might be supposed, therefore, that we need to claim either that such a human being is not a person with rights or has a low "quality of life" in some other sense, in order to justify this nearly universal conclusion. If so, this may constitute a serious challenge to the position I have taken on the framework in which these decisions must be made.

At this point we are faced with difficulties for which no easy answers seem to be available. If we believe intuitively that it may be proper to remove Miss Quinlan's respirator, then we must find a rationale for so doing that does not entail a fundamental break with the proper horizon within which these choices must be made. But if we exclude, as I think we must, appeals to Karen's low "quality of life," then it may appear difficult to offer another plausible rationale for such an action.

At this point there are two admittedly imperfect ways to approach such cases, which we touched briefly upon in chapter three. The first is to focus on the actual prognosis of the majority of patients in a persistent vegetative state. The available data show that most patients with permanent coma will not survive more than one year from the onset of the coma. The reasons for this seem to vary from patient to patient, often as the result of multiple, complex medical problems in the patient. Patients in a permanent coma are extremely susceptible to infection, which may not be controlled very well with available drugs. In other cases the source of the coma will be some underlying pathological process that itself is associated with a grim prognosis, such as hepatic coma resulting from liver failure. Finally, it may simply be that the brain is such a complex, interrelated mechanism that such damage as will be necessary to produce a persistent vegetative state will also affect the capacity of the organism to sustain life in so many subtle ways that prognosis for long term survival is rendered very uncertain in this respect.[40]

A second way to look at these cases is to say that the permanently comatose person has lost something that is essential as a prerequisite for one's having a right to life. If so, then removing one from artificial life-support would not constitute a moral or legal wrong to the person. If no harm were done to third parties and the risk of expanding the range of cases were foreclosed, then the act itself and a policy that permitted it would be acceptable.[41] On this view rights are connected to the potential capacity to experience the consequences of exercising the right in question. This does not mean that rights pertain to every possible experience; such a view was rejected earlier in this chapter. The point made here is that the capacity for experience may be a threshold for making a coherent claim of right. Human beings cannot be said to have fundamental rights to do that which human beings cannot do, such as travel to other galaxies. Human beings can coherently be said to have a right to the protection of their lives or the practice of religion because they can experience the exercise of such rights as "good."

In general this view is not objectionable when applied to the distinction between human beings and nonhuman animals or inanimate objects. The question is whether we can say that it applies to the possession of rights among human beings. In some sense the answer here seems to be yes. For example, the person who cannot even know what religions or churches are cannot really be said to be exercising a right of religious freedom or worship when one is taken to church. It does not even seem to be intelligible to claim otherwise. Such examples could be multiplied, but they all seem to come to the same point: the capacity to experience the results of exercising a right, such as religious worship, appears to be a threshold for a claim of rights.[42]

If this is a plausible way of looking at these cases, then the sentience standard noted in chapter three would be the appropriate standard for dealing with patients in a persistent vegetative state. If the patient had any sentience at all, then we could ascribe to him or her a right to life and if my argument is correct, quality-of-life judgments would be excluded at this point. If the patient is not sentient, then we would not violate any of his or her rights by removing artificial life supports. Since he or she is typically not in pain and cannot suffer, we would need strong independent reasons for a decision not to treat aggressively these patients. Such reasons might include the grief of the family or the declining prognosis of the patient but in so acting we would not, on this account be involved in a serious wrong *vis-á-vis* the patient.

This way of viewing these cases avoids the confusions and evasions resulting from the claim that comatose patients have rights that can be exercised for them by others. As we saw in the discussion of euthanasia, this position is taken in some leading court cases, but it is a transparently evasive maneuver, avoiding the plain quality-of-life judgment of the court and the family.

The question addressed by this view is a threshold question, not a quality-of-life judgment that could expand easily in the direction of the sentient but senile.

The resolution that I have offered to these cases of persons in a persistent vegetative state is tentative and imperfect. They are cases that test the limits of our collective theorizing; no solution is likely to be fully satisfying. My view has some affinity to that originally advanced by Paul Ramsey, though my argument is couched in the more political language of rights than in the language of care that he uses.[43]

Even though these are difficult cases where answers are elusive, we should not let such cases become the basis of a policy that would apply to a far broader range of persons with limited mental capacities—the retarded, the senile or demented, and so forth. The weakness of the other available alternatives we have seen throughout this book; we should seek a resolution to the case of patients in permanent coma that does not involve us in those alternatives.

This policy is not perfect. It is not meant to be. Nor can I claim that every conceivable case can be easily resolved in its terms.The complexities of clinical decision making are much too diverse to make any such claim seem plausible; but I do claim that in many cases this policy can produce a humane outcome which is plausible for contemporary practice.

No law or policy can produce certitude in our judgment or perfect justice in our actions. The limits of law and policy are reached when it has set forth the horizon within which the individual agent can evaluate one's acts and when it has excluded those actions and plans that debase justice. Law thus excludes the worst of our vices and behaviors but it does not offer us the salvific balm of absolute rectitude or justice.

Conclusion

The epigraph of this book and its title were taken from Dietrich Bonhoeffer, the German theologian executed by the Nazis for his participation in the plot against Hitler's life.[1] But this does not mean that this book is a religious tract. Indeed, Bonhoeffer believed that in a world come of age Christianity should be religionless—free of sectarian squabbles, and unobsessed by an otherworld, it should call humankind to the perfection of human justice and integrity. He believed in the essence of the liberal society in opposition with the tyranny he confronted.

The public life of liberal societies is premised on the belief in the intrinsic equal worth of each human life, irrespective of the qualities which it manifests. This does not mean that we are unmindful of the differences in various lives or the importance of such differences in various social matters. Even a brief acquaintance with the way that various welfare entitlements are based on the handicap of the recipient suggests otherwise. Nonetheless, the most enduring premise of our society, one coeval with its existence, is that such differences are not of ultimate significance; they do not mark the boundary of those who count as members of the community, entitled to its protection and generosity.

It is this conviction that is under assault today from those who assert that communal membership and the moral and legal standing it confers must be derived not from one simply being a human life, but from one's worth or qualities. In the various chapters of this book, we have seen how this view is being pressed with increasing vigor in several fields of medicine. Given their currency in contemporary medical and social dialogue, these arguments certainly deserve the treatment they have received here. At the same time, the serious problems we have noted in these claims should not obscure the larger view to which we have called attention throughout. In whatever form they are offered, these sorts of claims press on us a radically new horizon of thought, policy, and action. They do more than ask us to alter a somewhat awkward social policy; rather, they ask us to reshape our collective vision in fundamentally new ways. The shape of this new vision is such a departure from the horizon of choice that has heretofore formed us as a community that it can be classified as revolutionary in the fullest sense of the term. The full scope and meaning of this revolution are as yet unknown and its outcome is even more uncertain. Here we have been concerned to point out the nature of this revolution, and as much as can be said about the implications to which it seems to point.

In a much-neglected book, Sebastian de Grazia once wrote:

> The great community, as the ancient Greeks understood well, the community which embraces all other communities is the political community. Holding it together are systems of belief, flexible bands weaving through and around each member of the community, compacting it, allowing some stretch at times, coiling like a steel spring at others. The basic denominator of citizens is these belief systems which express their ideas concerning their relationship to one another and to their rulers. Without them, without this fundament of commonality, no political community can be said, to exist.[2]

This is the outlook that has informed both the critical and constructive parts of the inquiry that has gone before in this book. Individual acts of public decision and choice do not occur in a vacuum of spontaneous desire and will; they emerge in a community that is shaped by a specific horizon of choice, a community attached to a vision of the just and the good that gives meaning to the whole and illumines the ambiguities and shadows of civic life and choice.

None of this provides us with absolute certainty in our choices or perfection in our public norms. The limitations of human life are too much to expect any such perfection; those who have sought to find or apply in practice such a perfect master schema for decision and choice, from Bentham's utilitarianism to the various rule formalists in jurisprudence, have been completely disappointed.

In our own inquiries here, we have seen all too clearly the ambiguities of medical decision making in these most crucial areas, ambiguities that neither moral theory nor law and guidelines can resolve. To exclude from law and policy, and thus from the context of choice, judgments about the quality-of-life does not relieve us of the burdens of doubt or the perplexities of decision.

At the most it shapes our vision and orders the range of acceptable choices before us. This is not insignificant, for the permanence of our vision calls attention to our most central commitments as a people, ones that law must preserve and policy reflect.

Precisely in the commitment to equal worth, we have seen, do liberal societies distinguish themselves from the alternatives available and exclude from their midst those policies that are incompatible with this vision. Liberal societies deliberately found themselves on an abstraction from the question of the good for man as such and thus on an abstraction from what makes human life worthwhile or worthless. But without such knowledge in the definitive form of the divine or the godlike, we are confronted with the contradictory, confusing, and dangerously elastic formulations that we have seen throughout this book.

265

The great legal scholar Roscoe Pound once wrote that "law prevents the sacrifice of ultimate interests, social and individual, to the more obvious and pressing but less weighty immediate interests."[3] If this is true of all law, it is even more true of the fundamental principles that lie at the core of our common life together and are found frequently enunciated in constitutional texts. These principles set forth a vision of our ultimate commitments as citizens amid the flow of public desire and political pressure. In a very real sense, they define the essence of our life together as an organized political regime. Most especially, they give direction as to who counts as a member of this community and who is entitled to the minimal rights afforded to all such members equally.

I believe that, seen in this light, the contemporary debate over the various forms of abortion, euthanasia, and suicide and their potential enactment into law pose no less severe a test to our collective principles than did the slavery crisis that was confronted a century ago. To the extent that we come to the point in our law of allowing one person or group to decide that another human being ought to live no more, to that extent we will have granted that party the power to decide that another human being is no longer entitled to the most minimal of our civil rights. Have we not then allowed one human being to treat another as if he or she were not a human being at all in the most significant political sense—that is, a being endowed with certain inalienable rights?

Once we permit the freedom to choose for another or to endorse and support his choice to include the freedom to deny his civil equality we move in a direction that ends with the denial of freedom itself. Even Mill and Locke knew that the freedom to sell oneself into slavery, no matter how happy one might be enslaved, was the ultimate perversion of freedom. It may very well be that we are seeing another version of this same error among those who wish to endorse as a final solution to the problems of the weak, the suffering, and the helpless a policy that ends in claiming that some human lives are not worth protecting and sustaining anymore.

266

Notes

Introduction

1. Bonnie Steinbock, "Baby Jane Doe in the Courts," *Hastings Center Report* 14 (February 1984): 13–19; Marcia Chambers, "Baby Doe: Hard Case for Parents and Courts," *New York Times* January 8, 1984; State of New York, Court of Appeals, Brief for Petitioner—Appelant (hereafter Appelant's Brief); Court of Appeals, Brief for Respondents, Stony Brook Hospital and the State University of New York at Stony Brook (hereafter Respondent's Brief).

2. Appelant's Brief, 11–13; Respondent's Brief, 2; Steinbock, "Baby Jane Doe in the Courts," 14.

3. David McClone and James Brown, "Treatment Choices for the Infant with Meningomyelocele," in D. Horan and M. Delahoyde, eds. *Infanticide and the Handicapped Newborn* (Provo, Utah: Brigham Young University Press, 1982), 69–75.

4. Steinbock, "Baby Jane Doe in the Courts," 14; Appelant's Brief, 10–11; *Weber* v. *Stony Brook Hospital*, State of New York, Supreme Court, Appelate Division, October 21, 1983.

5. Appelant's Brief, 10; transcript, *People ex rel Washburn* v. *Stony Brook Hospital*, State of New York, Supreme Court, October 19, 1983, 46.

6. Transcript, *People ex rel Washburn* v. *Stony Brook Hospital*, State of New York, Supreme Court, October 19, 1983, 26, 179.

7. Steinbock, "Baby Jane Doe in the Courts," 14, repeats this confusion about a small head as does *New York Times*, January 8, 1984.

8. Transcript, 44.

9. Transcript, 141, and especially the interview with Dr. Butler in the November 9, 1983 issue of *Newsday*, which repeats much of his optimistic assessment of Baby Jane.

10. McLone's evaluation, based on the trial transcript, is contained in a press release from Americans United for Life, December 5, 1983.

11. *New York Times*, October 21, 1983.

12. *Weber* v. *Stony Brook Hospital*, State of New York, Supreme Court, Appelate Division, 489 N.E. 2d 1193.

13. *Weber* v. *Stony Brook Hospital*, New York State, Court of Appelate, October 28, 1983; 490 N.E. 2d 481.

14. *New York Times*, November 2, 1983; section 504 is found at 29 US Code 794 and its implementing regulations are at 45 Code of Federal Regulations par. 80.6.

15. *United States of America* v. *Stony Brook Hospital*, United States District Court, Eastern District of New York, 575 F. Supp 607, 1983.

16. *United States of America* v. *Stony Brook Hospital*, United States Court of Appeals, 2nd. Circuit, 729 F. 2d 144.

17. George Annas, "When Suicide Prevention Becomes Brutality," *Hastings Center Report* 14 (April 1984): 20–22; *New York Times*, October 30, 1983.

18. Annas, "When Suicide Prevention Becomes Brutality," 21; *New York Times*, November 3, November 4, 1983.

19. *New York Times*, December 6, 7, 8, 9, 1983; *Bouvia* v. *County of Riverside*, Superior Court, County of Riverside, California, December 16, 1983.

20. *New York Times*, September 18, 20, 22, 30, 1983.

21. *New York Times*, November 8, 1983.

22. These cases are treated in more detail in chapter three.

23. For a brief review of these cases, see Robert Veatch, *Death, Dying and the Biological Revolution* (New Haven: Yale University Press, 1976).

24. Roscoe Pound, "Justice According to Law," *Columbia Law Review* 13 (1913): 706.

Chapter One: *Political Regimes and Public Policies*

1. Plato, *The Republic*, trans. Allan Bloom (New York: Basic Books, 1968).

2. *Republic*, 543a–592b, 221–75.

3. See especially Leo Strauss, *Natural Right and History* (Chicago: University of Chicago Press, 1953); and Leo Strauss, *The City and Man* (Chicago: Rand MacNally, 1964).

4. This point can be documented in any of the standard textbooks on ethics currently in use. For examples, one can see Richard Brandt, *Ethical Theory* (Englewood Cliffs; Prentice Hall, 1959) and William Frankena, *Ethics* (Englewood Cliffs: Prentice Hall, 1964); for a brilliant discussion of the way specific moral problems or quandaries become the point of reference in ethical reflection, from which general rules are supposed to be constructed, see Edmund Pincoffs, "Quandary Ethics," *Mind* 80 (1971): 552–71.

5. The essential text in this regard is Plato's *Apology*, in which the inability of the city to take account of Socrates is the essential point. See also Strauss, *The City and Man*.

6. For examples, see Cicero, *Republic*, trans. C. W. Keyes. (Cambridge: Harvard University Press, 1928), book 1; Al-Farabi, *The Political Regime*, in M. Mahdi and R. Lerner, ed. *Medieval Political Philosophy* (New York: The Free Press, 1962), 31–57; Thomas Aquinas, *Summa Theologiae*, I-II, qq. 96–106.

7. Plato, *Laws*, trans. Thomas Pangle (New York: Basic Books, 1979), 873c.

8. Peter Peterson, "The Coming Crash of Social Security," *New York Review of Books* 29 (December 4, 1982): 34–39; Eli Ginzberg, "The Social Security System," *Scientific American* 246 (January 1982), 51–57; Stephen Crystal, *America's Old Age Crisis* (New York: Basic Books, 1982).

9. Peter Peterson, "The Salvation of Social Security," *New York Review of Books* 29 (December 16, 1982): 50–57; *Social Security in America's Future: The Final Report of the National Commission on Social Security* (Washington D.C.: US Government Printing Office, 1982).

10. J. G. Anderson, "Demographic Factors Affecting Health Services Utilization," *Medical Care* 11 (1973): 104–20; Paul Feldstein, *Health Care Economics* (New York: John Wiley, 1982).

11. John Hinton, *Dying* (London: Penguin Books, 1972), 80–82; R. Schulz, "Effects of Control and Predictability on the Physical and Psychological Well Being of the Aged," *Journal of Personality and Social Psychology* 33 (1976): 563–73.

12. Strauss, *The City and Man,* 136–40. See also Joseph Cropsey, "The United States as a Regime and the Sources of the American Way of Life," in Robert Horwitz, ed., *The Moral Foundations of the American Republic* (Charlottesville, Va.: University of Virginia Press, 1977), 86–101.

13. Jean-Jacques Rousseau, *The Government of Poland,* trans. F. Watkins (New York: Nelson, 1953); see also Cicero, *Republic* 1:47; 5:5–7, and *Laws* 1:14–176; Al-Farabi, *The Political Regime* and *The Attainment of Happiness.*

14. See Roger Barrus, "The Mormon Founding of Utah," unpublished Ph. D. dissertation, Harvard University, 1984.

15. This description applies to traditional Shiite Islam, not other branches of the faith. These differences are not germane here.

16. Wilmore Kendall, "The Open Society and Its Fallacies," *American Political Science Review* 54 (1960): 972–79. See also Rousseau, *Letter to D'Alembert* and *Social Contract;* on the latter I have learned much from Hilail Gildin, *Rousseau's Social Contract* (Chicago: University of Chicago Press, 1983); see also Thomas Jefferson, *Notes on the State of Virginia,* ed. William Peden (Chapel Hill: University of North Carolina Press, 1955), where a diversity of fundamental political opinions is held not to be good.

17. See especially Karl Popper, *The Open Society and Its Enemies* 2 vols. (London: Oxford University Press, rev. ed. 1961).

18. In his classic treatise, *On Liberty,* John Stewart Mill seems to reject this common view of liberalism. His analysis, however, is seriously flawed by his facile assumptions concerning the rationality or reasonableness of the citizens of his "open society." His essay does not treat passion and self-interest, does not admit that passion often triumphs over reason, that factions form in defiance of truth and that, once formed, no amount of evidence will dissuade the bigot from his or her cherished prejudices. All of these issues were central concerns of most other liberal theorists, especially those who concerned them-

selves with the actual governance of a free society. Confer Alexander Hamilton, James Madison, John Jay, *The Federalist* (Middletown, Conn.: Wesleyan University Press, 1961), especially number 10, and Rousseau, *Letter to D'Alembert*.

19. The essential works here are those of David Easton: *The Political System* (Chicago: University of Chicago Press, second edition, 1981) and *A Systems View of Political Life* (Chicago: University of Chicago Press, 1965, revised edition, 1979).

20. *The Politics of Aristotle*, ed. and trans. Ernest Barker (New York: Oxford University Press, 1949), Preface, lxvi; 1278b and the following.

21. *Politics of Aristotle*, 1280a–81a.

22. *Politics of Aristotle*, 1290a.

23. *Politics of Aristotle*, 1292a.

24. *Politics of Aristotle*, 1286a. Here Aristotle discusses the relation of monarchy and the rule of law. One can also note the similar teaching in Plato, *Statesman*, 300 and the following.

25. *Politics of Aristotle*, 1292a–93; also 1287, on the relation of law and limited political rule.

26. *Politics of Aristotle*, 1287a.

27. *Nichomachean Ethics*, 1137a–38a; *Rhetoric*, 1373b.

28. *Politics of Aristotle*, 1290a.

29. *Rhetoric*, 1373a–74b.

30. *Politics of Aristotle*, 1284a.

31. *Politics of Aristotle*, 1302a–16b.

32. *Politics*, 1269b–71b.

33. Alexis de Tocqueville, *Democracy in America*, trans. George Lawrence (New York: Harper and Row, 1966).

34. De Tocqueville, *Democracy in America*, 1:1:8; 1:2:5; 1:2:9.

35. De Tocqueville, *Democracy in America*, 1:2:9; 2:1:5; 2:2:9.

36. De Tocqueville, *Democracy in America*, 1:2:9.

37. De Tocqueville, *Democracy in America*, 2:1:7; 2:2:5; 2:2:9.

38. De Tocqueville, *Democracy in America*, 1:2:5; 2:1:6.

39. De Tocqueville, *Democracy in America*, 2:1:5.

40. De Tocqueville, *Democracy in America*, 1:2:9.

41. De Tocqueville, *Democracy in America*, 2:1:5.

42. De Tocqueville, *Democracy in America*, 2:1:5; see also 1:2:5.

43. "The religious atmosphere of the country was the first thing that struck me on arrival in the United States." 1:2:9.

44. De Tocqueville, *Democracy in America*, 2:1:2; 1:2:9.

45. De Tocqueville, *Democracy in America*, 2:1:5.

46. De Tocqueville, *Democracy in America*, 1:1:3. De Tocqueville's general argument concerning the leveling of religious opinion in America and its importance in the American regime has been given a brilliant restatement in Will Herberg, *Protestant, Catholic, Jew* (New York: Doubleday, 1960).

47. More complete references on this point are found in the notes to chapter two, but the essential text for this view of politics is Locke's *Letter on Toleration*.

48. Rousseau, *Emile*, ed. Alan Bloom (New York: Basic Books, 1980), book 4. In the final sections of *Emile*, Rousseau tries to show how education can moderate the tensions between compassion and acquisitiveness.

Chapter Two: *Liberal Polities*

1. See Leo Strauss, *Natural Right and History;* Roberto Ungar, *Knowledge and Politics* (New York: Free Press, 1975).

2. Strauss, *Natural Right and History.*

3. *Statesman,* 300d.

4. See Thomas Hobbes, *Leviathan,* ed. M. Oakeshott (London: Collier Books, 1962) 2:17–19; Locke, *Two Treatises,* ed. Peter Laslett (Cambridge: Cambridge University Press, 1960), 2:7–9; Rousseau, *The Social Contract,* book 1; especially Spinoza, *The Political Treatise,* chapter 1, where the truth about politics is said to be found by viewing man as ruled by passions and vices.

5. John Rawls, *A Theory of Justice* (Cambridge: Harvard University Press, 1971), 315–22, 527.

6. On Rawls, see Vinit Haksar, *Equality, Liberty and Perfectionism,* "Clarendon Library of Logic and Philosophy," (Oxford: Oxford University Press, 1979).

7. For the rest, see Claes Ryn, *Democracy and the Ethical Life* (Baton Rouge: Louisiana State University Press, 1976).

8. Strauss, *Natural Right and History,* and Leo Strauss, *Liberalism: Ancient and Modern* (New York: Free Press, 1963); also see Locke, *Two Treatises* 2:8, paragraph 95 ff.

9. Spinoza, for example, articulated a thoroughly subjectivist account of morality in his *Ethics,* an account that figures prominently in his political philosophy. In both his *Theological-Political Treatise* and his unfinished *Political Treatise,* he portrays the ruler as constrained by the rule of law precisely because man is always a slave to passion and thus moral knowledge of the constant sort required for governance is impossible. In the long run, it is safer to have the rule of law than the rule of passion. See Spinoza, *Ethics,* trans. R. H. Elwes (New York: Dover Books, 1951), part 4; *Theological-Political Treatise,* trans. R. H. Elwes (New York: Dover Books, 1951), chapter 16; and especially the discussion of Spinoza in Richard Popkin, *The History of Skepticism from Erasmus to Spinoza* (Berkeley: University of California Press, 2nd edition, 1979).

10. Harvey Mansfield, "Thomas Jefferson," in Morton Frisch and Richard Stevens, eds., *American Political Thought* (New York: Scribners, 1970).

11. Locke, *Second Treatise,* 2:5.

12. Hooker, *Laws of Ecclesiastical Polity,* 1:8, paragraph 7.

13. Locke, *Second Treatise* 2:7–10.

14. Locke, *Second Treatise,* 2:5.

15. Locke, *Second Treatise,* 2:8.

16. Hobbes, *Leviathan* c. 38.

17. Hobbes, *Leviathan* c. 38.

18. Hobbes, *Leviathan,* c. 38.

19. Also see Immanuel Kant, "On the Common Saying: This may be True in Theory but does not Apply in Practice," section 2, in *Kant's Political Texts,* ed. H. Reiss (Cambridge: Cambridge University Press, 1970).

20. See Mansfield, "Thomas Jefferson."

21. Harry Jaffa, *How to Think About the American Revolution* (Durham, N.C.: Carolina Academic Press, 1977); Harry Jaffa, *Equality and Liberty* (New York: Oxford University Press, 1963).

22. John Rawls, *Theory of Justice*, 504–12.

23. L. Koppleman, "Respect and the Retarded," in L. Koppleman and J. Moskop, eds., *Ethics and Mental Retardation* (Boston: D. Reidel, 1984), 65–85.

24. B. Williams, "The Idea of Equality," in P. Laslett and W. G. Runciman, eds., *Philosophy, Politics and Society*, 2nd Series, (London: Barnes and Noble, 1961), 39–60. For a trenchant defense of Williams, see Amy Gutman, *Democratic Equality* (New York: Oxford University Press, 1979). It should be noted that Gutman in particular is most concerned with economic inequality and inequality in representation and thus can glide over the foundational questions we are raising. For an excellent discussion of the character of equality as a postulate in liberal theory, see William Blackstone, "The Meaning and Character of the Equality Principle," *Ethics* 77 (1967): 239–53.

25. On the political primacy of the needs of the body, the essential text is John Locke, *Letter on Toleration*, 170–75. Rawls's theory of primary goods is almost a lineal descendant of Locke's notion of civic goods. See Rawls, *A Theory of Justice*, 90–95.

26. James Wilson, *Works*, ed. Robert McClosky 2 vols. (Cambridge: Harvard University Press, 1967), 1:241.

27. The most trenchant presentation of this view is Michael Tooley, *Abortion and Infanticide* (New York: Oxford University Press, 1983).

28. Tooley, *Abortion and Infanticide*, 303–60.

29. This would be a view of "mental state" that would surely find favor in much of post-Witgensteinian philosophy, especially philosophy of mind. Furthermore, the notion that cognitive mental states are the key to personal identity, as Tooley seems to suppose, has not gone unchallenged. See especially D. M. Rosenthal, "Emotions and the Self," in K. D. Irani and G. E. Meyers, editors, *Emotion: Philosophical Studies* (New York: Haven Publishing, 1983), 164–91.

30. This whole connection between rights and interests or desires has been strenuously attacked from the point of view of moral theory in Philip Devine, *The Ethics of Homicide* (Ithaca: Cornell University Press, 1978).

31. Hobbes, *Leviathan*, c. 18; Locke, *Second Treatise*, paragraphs 124–31; Rousseau, *The Social Contract* is another essential text in this regard. For an interesting discussion of some of the problems of representative government as well as a very thorough bibliography,

see Hanna Pitkin, *The Concept of Representation* (Berkeley: University of California Press, 1972).

32. See especially here Gary Glenn, "Abortion and Inalienable Rights in Classical Liberalism," *American Journal of Jurisprudence* 20 (1975): 62–80; Gary Glenn, "Hobbes on Inalienable Rights," paper given at the International Hobbes Tercentenary Conference, Boulder, Colorado, August 1979. Also see A. Kuflik, "The Inalienability of Autonomy," *Philosophy and Public Affairs* (1984) 13:270–98. Kuflik seems to miss much of the political context and meaning of the notion of inalienable rights in classical liberalism.

33. Hobbes, *Leviathan*, chapter 14.

34. One can document this for oneself in Plato, Aristotle, Xenophon, Cicero, and countless medieval thinkers such as al-Farabi and Thomas Aquinas. For an introduction to the issues, see Leo Strauss, *On Tyranny* (Ithaca: Cornell University Press, 1963).

35. Glenn, "Hobbes on Inalienable Rights."

36. *Republic*, 460c. Infanticide was widely practiced in the ancient world, and is noted by many sources such as Herodotus, Strabo, and Aristotle. Most of the relevant texts are brought together in W. L. Newman, ed., *The Politics of Aristotle: With an Introduction, Notes and Essays* (Oxford: The Clarendon Press, 1902), 3:473–75.

37. Plato, *Laws*, 864b–974.

38. William Blackstone, *Commentary on the Laws of England*, ed. W. G. Hammond (San Francisco: Bancroft and Whithey, 1890), 1:9 ff.

39. See Roberto Ungar, *Law in Modern Society* (New York: Free Press, 1975).

40. See Sir John Fortescue, *The Governance of England*, (Westport, Conn.: Hyperion Press, 1979), 3; Sir Henry de Bracton, *On the Laws and Customs of England*, trans. Samuel E. Thorne (Cambridge: Harvard University Press, 1969) 2:253–55; and the various formulations in Edward Coke which approach modern notions of the idea. Also see Sir William Holdsworth, *A History of English Law* (London: Methuen, 1924), 10:647–50.

41. See Plato, *Statesman*, 300 ff; Spinoza, *Political Treatise*, chapters 6–7.

42. Locke, *Two Treatises*, 2:19, section 219.

43. See Ungar, *Law in Modern Society*, 167–70, where the imperfections of impersonal rules are trenchantly noted.

44. Edward Kennedy, "Toward a New System of Criminal Sentencing: Law with Order," *American Criminal Law Review* (1979) 16:353–83. M. Frankel, *Criminal Sentencing* (New York: Hill and Wang, 1975).

45. C. Thomas and W. A. Fitch, "The Exercise of Discretionary Decision Making by the Police," *North Dakota Law Review* 54 (1977): 61–98.

46. See chapter five below.

47. Germain Grisez and Joseph Boyle, *Life and Death with Liberty and Justice* (South Bend: University of Notre Dame Press, 1979), 131–34.

48. See *Abraham Lincoln: His Speeches and Writings*, ed. Roy Basler (Cleveland: World Publishing Co., 1946), 401–3; Herbert Storing, "Slavery and the Constitution," in Robert Horwitz, ed., *The Moral Foundations of the American Republic* (Charlottesville: University of Virginia Press, 1977).

49. Lincoln passionately believed that the existence of slavery on American soil was ultimately incompatible with the essence of a regime founded on the principles articulated in the *Declaration of Independence;* see Lincoln, "Speeches and Writings, 372–81—his famous "Springfield Address of 1858"—and his reply to Douglas in the seventh debate in *The Lincoln-Douglas Debates,* ed. R. W. Johanson (New York: Oxford University Press, 1965), 307; also see Harry Jaffa, *Crisis of the House Divided* (New York: Doubleday, 1959).

50. Lincoln, "Speech at Columbus, Ohio, September 1859," in *In the Name of the People*, ed. Harry Jaffa and R. W. Johanson (Columbus: Ohio State University Press, 1959), 267–68.

51. Lincoln, "Speech at Columbus, Ohio, September 1859," 269.

52. For Douglas's view, see his famous essay "Popular Sovereignty in the Territories," reprinted in Jaffa and Johanson, eds., *In the Name of the People,* 58–125. Also see Jaffa, *Crisis of the House Divided,* 104–79.

53. Jaffa and Johanson, eds., *In the Name of the People,* 55. Also see Lincoln's "Speech at Cincinnati September 1859," reprinted in this same collection.

54. John Robertson, "Involuntary Euthanasia of Defective Newborns," *Stanford Law Review* 27 (1975): 213–69.

Chapter Three: *Infanticide*

1. John Robertson, "Involuntary Euthanasia of Defective Newborns;" 213–67; Philip Heymann and Sarah Holtz, "The Severely Defective Newborn: The Dilemma and the Decision Process," *Public Policy* 23 (1975): 381–417.

2. William Langer, "Checks on Population Growth: 1750–1850," *Scientific American* 226 (February 1982): 92–99; Barbara Kellum, "Infanticide in England in the Later Middle Ages," *History of Childhood Quarterly* 1 (1974): 367–78; R. H. Helmholtz, "Infanticide in the Province of Canterbury in the Fifteenth Century," *History of Childhood Quarterly* 1 (1974): 379–90.

3. George Behlmer, "Deadly Motherhood: Infanticide and Medical Opinion in Mid-Victorian England," *Journal of the History of Medicine* 35 (1979): 403–27.

4. Catherine Damme, "Infanticide: The Worth of an Infant Under Law," *Medical History* 22 (1978): 1–24.

5. See Oscar Werner, *The Unmarried Mother in German Literature* (New York: Columbia University Press, 1917); J. A. Easton, *Contributions to Legal Medicine: Being Observations on the Jurisprudence of Infanticide* (Edinburgh: Sutherland and Fox, 1852).

6. John Freemen, "Is There a Right to Die—Quickly?" *Journal of Pediatrics* 80 (1972): 904–8.

7. The literature here is vast and only a few key titles can be noted. See Raymond Duff and A. G. Campbell, "Moral and Ethical Dilemmas in the Special Care Nursery," *New England Journal of Medicine* 189 (1973): 890–94; John Fletcher, "Abortion, Euthanasia and Care of Defective Newborns," *The New England Journal of Medicine* 292 (1975): 75–78; John Paris, "Terminating Treatment for Newborns: A Theological Perspective," *Law Medicine and Health Care* 12 (1982): 120–24; Anthony Shaw, "Dilemmas of Informed Consent in Children," *New England Journal of Medicine* 289 (1973): 885–89; G. K. Smith and E. D. Smith, "Selection for Treatment in Spina Bifida Cystica," *British Medical Journal* 4 (1973): 189–93.

Good collections of papers on these issues are contained in five works: Dennis Horan and Melinda Delhoyde, eds., *Infanticide and the Handicapped Newborn* (Provo: Brigham Young University Press, 1982); Albert Johnson and Michael Garland, eds., *Ethics of Newborn Intensive Care* (Berkeley: Institute of Governmental Studies, University of California, 1976); Marvin Kohl, ed., *Infanticide and the Value of Life* (Buffalo:

Prometheus Books, 1979); Chester Swinyard, ed., *Decision Making and the Defective Newborn* (Springfield: Charles Thomas, 1978); R. Weir, *Selective Non-Treatment of Handicapped Newborns* (New York: Oxford University Press, 1984).

8. Donald Matson, "Surgical Treatment of Myelomeningocele," *Pediatrics* 42 (1968): 225.

9. H. T. Englehardt, "Euthanasia and Children: The Injury of Continued Existence," *Journal of Pediatrics* 83 (1973): 70–71; H. T. Englehardt, "Aiding the Death of Young Children," in Marvin Kohl, ed., *Beneficient Euthanasia* (Buffalo: Prometheus Books, 1973), 180–92.

10. Richard Brandt, "Defective Newborns and the Morality of Termination," in Kohl, ed., *Infanticide,* 46–57.

11. Brandt, "Defective Newborns and the Morality of Termination," 49.

12. J. Lorber, "Results of Treatment of Myeolomeningocele," *Developmental Medicine and Child Neurology* 13 (1971): 279–303.

13. This point about exceptions to rules is explored in a very different context in Marcus Singer, *Generalization in Ethics* (New York: Alfred Knopf, 1961), 75–90, and in Paul Ramsey, "The Case of the Curious Exception," in Paul Ramsey and Gene Outka, eds., *Norm and Context in Christian Ethics* (New York: Charles Scribners, 1967), 67–135.

14. Raymond Duff, "On Deciding the Use of the Family Commons," *Birth Defects: Original Article Series* 12 (1976): 73–84; Raymond Duff, "On Deciding the Care of Severely Handicapped or Dying Persons," *Pediatrics* 37 (1976): 487–92. This view is also partially endorsed in the report of the President's Commission for the Study of Ethical Problems in Medicine and Biomedical and Behavioral Research, *Deciding to Forego Life Sustaining Treatment* (Washington, D.C. US Government Printing Office, 1983), 197–228. Available survey data shows that the wishes of the family are crucial in the decision-making process.

15. Norman Fost, "Counseling Families Who Have a Child with a Severe Congenital Anomaly," *Pediatrics* 67 (1981): 321–24; E. D'Arcy, "Congenital Defect: Mothers' Reactions to First Information," *British Medical Journal* 3 (1968): 796–800; N. Johns, "Family Reactions to the Birth of a Child with a Congenital Anomaly," *Medical Journal of Australia* 5 (1971): 277–81.

16. The available survey data shows a remarkable consistency in following parental wishes. See "Treating the Defective Newborn: A Survey of Physicians' Attitudes," *Hastings Center Reports* 6 (1976): 2–5; A. Shaw et al., "Ethical Issues in Pediatric Surgery: A National Survey," *Pediatrics* 60 (1977): 588–92.

17. See G. H. Zuk, "The Religious Factor and Role of Guilt in Parental Acceptance of the Retarded Child," *American Journal of Mental Deficiencies* 64 (1959): 145–53, and B. Farber et al., "Family Background and the Decision to Have a Retarded Child," in Swinyard, ed., *Decision Making and the Defective Newborn*, 193–245.

18. More than a hundred years of legal development is unanimous in the conclusion that a parent may not refuse clearly life-saving treatment for his or her child. For examples, see *People ex rel Wallace* v. *Labrenz* 104 N.E. 2d 759 (1952); *Morrison* v. *State* 252 S.W. 2d 97 (1952); *Hoener* v. *Bertinato* 171 A. 2d. 140 (1961); *In re Clark* 185 N.E. 2d 128 (1962); *In re Vasko* 263 N.Y.S. 522 (1933); *State* v. *Perricone* 181 A. 2d 751 (1961); *People* v. *Pierson* 68 N.E. 243 (1903). For a review of cases and issues, see Robertson, "Involuntary Euthanasia of Defective Newborns."

19. Terrence Ackerman, "Myelomeningocele and Parental Commitment: A Policy Proposal Regarding Selection for Treatment," *Man and Medicine* 5 (1980): 291–303.

20. Carson Strong, "Defective Infants and Their Impact on Families: Ethical and Legal Considerations," *Law Medicine and Health Care* 13 (1983): 10–15, and Carson Strong, "The Neonatologist's Duty to Patient and Parents," *Hasting Center Report* 14 (August 1984): 10–16.

21. See Richard McCormick, "Notes on Moral Theology," *Theological Studies* 44 (1983): 119–22.

22. See Warren Reich, "Quality of Life and Defective Newborn Children," in Swinyard, ed., *Decision Making and the Defective Newborn*, 489–511.

23. Marvin Kohl, "Voluntary Death and Meaningless Existence," in Kohl, ed., *Infanticide*, 210–11.

24. N. Robinson and H. Robinson, *The Mentally Retarded Child* (New York: McGraw Hill, 1976).

25. Kohl, "Voluntary Death and Meaningless Existence," 211.

26. See Paul Ramsey, *Ethics at the Edges of Life* (New York: Columbia University Press, 1978), and especially the critical essay by Peter

Singer, "President Reagan and Baby Doe," *New York Review of Books* (March 9, 1984).

27. See D. Walton, *On Death and Dying* (Montreal: McGill–Queens University Press, 1979).

28. D. Bakan, *Disease, Pain and Sacrifice* (Chicago: University of Chicago Press, 1968); D. Boeyink, "Pain and Suffering," *Journal of Religious Ethics* 2 (1974): 85–98; A. Petrie, *Individuality in Pain and Suffering* (Chicago: University of Chicago Press, 1967); V. D. Stravino, "The Nature of Pain," *Archives of Physical Medicine* 51 (1970): 37–44.

29. For a thorough review of the matter of brain death, see President's Commission, *Defining Death* (Washington, D.C.: US Government Printing Office, 1981).

30. Eric Cassel, "The Nature of Suffering and the Goals of Medicine," *New England Journal of Medicine* 306 (1982): 639–45.

31. Lorber, "Results of Treatment of Myelomeningocele"; B. Wright, *Physical Disability: A Psychological Approach* (New York: Harper and Row, 1960).

32. Joseph Fletcher, "Indicators of Humanhood," *Hastings Center Report* 2 (1972): 1–4.

33. The literature advocating such a view is vast; some examples are Kohl, ed., *Infanticide;* A. Jonson and M. Garland, "A Moral Policy for the Life/Death Decisions in the Intensive Care Nursery," in Jonson and Garland, eds., *Ethics of Newborn Intensive Care,* 142–55; John Paris, "Terminating Treatment for Newborns: A Theological Perspective," *Law, Medicine and Health Care* 12 (1982): 120–24.

34. Richard McCormick, "To Save or Let Die," *Journal of the American Medical Association* 229 (1974): 172–76; Richard McCormick, "A Proposal for Quality of Life Criteria for Sustaining Life," *Hospital Progress* 59 (1975): 76–79.

35. John Arras, "Towards an Ethic of Ambiguity," *Hastings Center Report* 14 (April 1984): 24–33.

36. Jonson and Garland, " Moral Policy for Life/Death Decisions," 142–55.

37. See 96–101.

38. Jonson and Garland, "Moral Policy for Life/Death Decisions," 148.

39. Raymond Duff and A. G. M. Campbell, "Authors' Response," *Journal of Medical Ethics* 5 (1979): 141–42.

40. For one statement of this view, see Carson Strong, "Positive Killing and the Permanently Unconscious Patient," *Bioethics Quarterly* 3 (1981): 190–205.

41. Leonard Weber, *Who Shall Live* (New York: Paulist Press, 1976), 93.

42. Benedict Ashley and Kevin O'Rourke, *Health Care Ethics* (St. Louis, Mo.: Catholic Health Association, 1982), 381–88.

43. Richard McCormick, "The Quality of Life, the Sanctity of Life," *Hastings Center Report* 8 (February 1978): 30–36.

44. Weber, *Who Shall Live*, 95.

45. Lorber, "Results of Treatment of Myelomeningocele," 300.

46. See also Ashley and O'Rourke, *Health Care Ethics*, 383.

47. For descriptions of the case, see Anne Bannion, M.D., "The Bloomington Baby," *Human Life Review* 7 (Fall, 1982): 3–10; "In the Matter of the Treatment and Care of Infant Doe: Declaratory Judgment," *Connecticut Medicine* 47 (1983): 409–10; Robert Weir, *Selective Non-Treatment of Handicapped Newborns* (New York: Oxford University Press, 1984), 128–29.

48. United States Code 974.

49. Notice of Interim Final Rule, Office of the Secretary, Department of Health and Human Services, "Non-Discrimination on the Basis of Handicap," 48 *Federal Register* 9630 (March 7, 1983).

50. See the data in H. J. Aaron and W. B. Schwartz, *The Painful Prescription* (Washington, D.C.: Brookings Institution, 1984).

51. Federal Register 9631 (March 7, 1983).

52. Norman Fost, "Putting Hospitals on Notice," *Hastings Center Reports* 12 (August 1982): 5–8; see also John Arras and Nancy Rhoden, "Withholding Treatment From Baby Doe," *Millbank Memorial Fund Quarterly* 63 (1985): 18–51.

53. *American Academy of Pediatrics* v. *Heckler* 561 F. Supp. 395 (1983).

54. Louisiana Revised Statutes 40.1299.36; Arizona Revised Statutes 13–3620; Indiana Revised Statutes 31.207.

55. Louisiana Revised Statutes 40.1299.36.

56. Louisiana Revised Statutes 40.1299.36.

57. Only a few titles can be cited: M. Angell, "Handicapped Children: Uncle Sam and Baby Doe," *New England Journal of Medicine*

309 (1983): 659–61; C. L. Bersath, "A Neonatalogist Looks at the Baby Doe Rule," *Pediatrics* 72 (1983): 429; John Connery, "An Analysis of the HHS Notice on Treating the Handicapped," *Hospital Progress* 62 (1982): 18–20; K. O'Rourke, "Lessons from the Infant Doe Case," *Connecticut Medicine* 47 (1983): 411–12; R. S. Shapiro, "Medical Treatment of Defective Newborns," *Harvard Journal on Legislation* 20 (1983): 137–52; S. Taub, "Medical Decisionmaking for Defective Infants," *Connecticut Medicine* 47 (1983): 413–16; R. F. Weir, "The Government and Selective Non-Treatment of Handicapped Infants," *New England Journal of Medicine* 309 (1983): 661–63.

58. See "Statement of the AMA to DHHS: Handicapped Infants," *Connecticut Medicine* 47 (1983): 417–20.

59. See *AAP* v. *Heckler;* Committee on Bioethics, American Academy of Pediatrics, "Treatment of Critically Ill Newborns," *Pediatrics* 72 (1983): 565–66; *United States of America* v. *Stony Brook Hospital;* Rhoden and Arras, "Withholding Treatment From Baby Doe," *Millbank Memorial Fund Quarterly* 63 (1985): 18–51.

60. DHHS, Office of Human Development Services, "Final Rule," 50 Federal Register 14878 (April 15, 1985).

61. DHHS, Office of Human Development Services, "Model Guidelines for Health Care Providers to Establish Infant Care Review Committees," 50 Federal Register 14893 (April 15, 1985).

62. See the discussion in chapter seven, 243–48.

Chapter Four: *Euthanasia*

1. For the last century the literature is vast. Useful bibliographic help may be found in Charles Triche and Diane Triche, *The Euthanasia Controversy 1812–1974: A Bibliography* (Troy, N.Y.: Whiston Publications, 1975); O. R. Russel, *Freedom to Die* (New York: Human Sciences Press, 1975). For journalist treatments, see Richard Trubo, *Act of Mercy* (Los Angeles: Nash, 1973); Marya Mannes, *Last Rights* (New York: Signet, 1975). For the legal problems, see Richard Sherlock, "The Right to Die as Public Policy: A Review," *Political Science Reviewer* 10 (1982): 251–86. For the viewpoints of philosophers and theologians, see Marvin Kohl, ed., *Beneficient Euthanasia* (Buffalo: Prometheus Books, 1975); Sissela Bok and John Behenke, ed., *Dilemmas of Euthanasia* (New York: Doubleday Anchor, 1975); A. B. Downing, ed., *Euthanasia and the Right to Die* (London: Peter Owen, 1969); David Hall

and Dennis Moran, eds., *Death, Dying and Euthanasia* (Baltimore: University Publications, 1975); John Ladd, ed., *Ethical Issues Relating to Life and Death* (New York: Oxford University Press, 1979.)

2. Alabama Code 22-31-1; Alaska Statutes 9.65.120; Arkansas Statutes Annotated 82-537; California Health and Safety Code 7180; Colorado Revised Statutes 12-36-136; Connecticut General Statutes Annotated 19-139; Florida Statutes 382-085; Georgia Code Annotated 88-1715; Hawaii Revised Statutes 327c-1; Idaho Code 54-1819; Illinois Statutes Annotated 302; Iowa Code Annotated 702.8; Kansas Statutes Annotated 77-202; Louisiana Code Annotated 14.15; Maryland Annotated Code 43.54; Michigan Statutes Annotated 14-15; Montana Revised Code Annotated 50-22-101; Nevada Revised Statutes 451.007; New Mexico Statutes Annotated 12-2-4; North Carolina General Statutes 90-323; Oklahoma Revised Statutes 1-301; Oregon Revised Statutes 146.087; Tennessee Code Annotated 53-459; Texas Revised Civil Statutes 4447t; Virginia Code 32-364.3.1; West Virginia Code 16-19; Wyoming Statutes 35-19-101.

3. Alabama Code 22-8-1; Arkansas Statutes Annotated 82-3801; California Health and Safety Code 7185; Delaware Code Annotated 16.2501; Idaho Code 39-4501; Kansas Statutes Annotated 65-28-101; Nevada Revised Statutes 449-510; New Mexico Statutes Annotated 24-7-1; North Carolina General Statutes 90-320; Oregon Revised Statutes 97.050; Texas Statutes Annotated 71-4590; Vermont Statutes Annotated 18.5251; Virginia Code 54-325.8; Washington Revised Code 70-122.

4. For a review of issues, statutes, and statutory proposals, see my essay "For Everything there is a Season: The Right to Die in American Law," *Brigham Young Law Review* No. 2 (1982): 545–616.

5. *In re Quinlan* 355 A.2d 647 (1976).

6. "Karen Ann Quinlan: A Family's Fate," *Washington Post*, 26 May 1981, 1.

7. D. Amundsen, "The Physician's Obligation to Prolong Life: A Medical Duty without Classical Roots," *Hastings Center Report* 8 (1978): 23–30; Stanley Reiser, "The Dilemma of Euthanasia in Modern Medical History," in Bok and Behenke, eds., *Dilemmas of Euthanasia.*

8. Hugh Trowell, *The Unfinished Debate on Euthanasia* (London: SCM Press, 1973).

9. Glanville Williams, *The Sanctity of Life and the Criminal Law* (New York: Alfred Knopf, 1957), 329–50. See the book reviews by

William Curran, *Harvard Law Review* 71 (1958): 585–89 and J. Donnelly, *Yale Law Journal* 67 (1958): 753–58; for an extended response, see Norman St. John Stevas, *Life, Death and the Law* (Bloomington: Indiana University Press, 1961).

10. See 149–51.

11. Williams, *The Sanctity of Life and the Criminal Law*, 318–33.

12. Williams, *The Sanctity of Life and the Criminal Law*, 311–19.

13. Williams, *The Sanctity of Life and the Criminal Law*, 333–50.

14. Williams, *The Sanctity of Life and the Criminal Law*, 333–50.

15. Yale Kamisar, "Some Non-Religious Views Against Proposed Mercy Killing Legislation," *Minnesota Law Review* 42 (1958): 969–1042.

16. Glanville Williams, "Mercy Killing Legislation—A Rejoinder," *Minnesota Law Review* 43 (1958): 37–56.

17. Kamisar, "Some Non-Religious Views Against Proposed Mercy Killing Legislation," 985–1013.

18. Kamisar, "Some Non-Religious Views Against Proposed Mercy Killing Legislation," 1015–41.

19. See Marvin Kohl, *The Morality of Killing* (New York: Humanities Press, 1974).

20. See Lon Fuller, *The Morality of Law* (New Haven: Yale University Press, 1968); Edwin Patterson, *Jurisprudence* (Brooklyn: Foundation Press, 1953), 96–116.

21. See James Rachels, "Euthanasia," in T. Regan, ed., *Matters of Life and Death* (New York: Random House, 1980).

22. Kohl, *The Morality of Killing*, 93; James Rachels, "Active and Passive Euthanasia," *New England Journal of Medicine* 292 (1975): 78–80; Michael Tooley, "An Irrelevant Consideration: Killing versus Letting Die," in B. Steinbock, ed., *Killing and Letting Die* (Englewood Cliffs: Prentice Hall, 1979), 56–63; Jonathan Glover, *Causing Death and Saving Lives* (London: Penguin, 1977).

23. Richard Trammel, "Saving Life and Taking Life," *Journal of Philosophy* 72 (1975): 131–37; Richard Trammel, "The Presumption against Taking Life," *Journal of Medicine and Philosophy* 3 (1978): 53–67; Paul Menzel, "Are Killing and Letting Die Morally Different in Medical Contexts?" *Journal of Medicine and Philosophy* 4 (1979): 269–93.

24. See H. L. A. Hart and A. M. Honoré, *Causation and the Law,* (Oxford: Clarendon Press, 1958).

25. In addition to the sources already noted, see Joseph Boyle, "Toward Understanding the Principle of the Double Effect," *Ethics* 90 (1980): 527–38; Germain Grisez, "Suicide and Euthanasia," in Horan and Mall, eds., *Death, Dying and Euthanasia,* 742–814; Joseph Boyle, "On Killing and Letting Die," *New Scholasticism* 51 (1977): 433–52.

26. Boyle, "Killing and Letting Die," 436.

27. See Philippa Foot, "The Problem of Abortion and the Doctrine of the Double Effect," *Oxford Review* 5 (1967): 5–15; A. Kenney, "Intention and Purpose in Law," in R. Summers, ed., *Essays in Legal Philosophy* (London: Oxford University Press, 1968), 146–63; R. A. Duff, "Absolute Principles and Double Effect," *Analysis* 36 (1976): 68–80.

28. Boyle, "Killing and Letting Die," 436.

29. *Dunlap* v. *United States* 70 F 2d 35 at 37; Restatement (second) of Law of Torts 8a (1965).

30. Perkins, *Criminal Law* (St. Paul, Minn.: West's Publishing Co., 1969), 747–50.

31. Boyle, "Killing and Letting Die," 436.

32. See Robert Burt, *Taking Care of Strangers* (New York: Free Press, 1979).

33. See Perkins, *Criminal Law,* 31; Herbert Weschler and Jerome Michael, "A Rationale for the Law of Homicide," *Columbia Law Review,* 37 (1937): 701; Williams, *The Sanctity of Life and the Criminal Law,* 318.

34. Robert Veatch, *Death, Dying and the Biological Revolution* (New Haven: Yale University Press, 1976); Norman Cantor, "A Patient's Decision to Refuse Life Saving Medical Care," *Rutgers Law Review,* 26 (1973): 228–64; Benedict Ashley and Kevin O'Rourke, *Health Care Ethics* (St. Louis: Catholic Health Association, 1982).

35. See Tom Beauchamp, "Euthanasia," in T. Regan, ed., *Matters of Life and Death,* 67–108.

36. Robert Byrn, "Compulsory Life-Saving Treatment for the Competent Adult," *Fordham Law Review* 44 (1975): 1–36.

37. Byrn, "Compulsory Life-Saving Treatment," 16–20.

38. George Fletcher, "Prolonging Life," *Washington Law Review* 42 (1967): 999–1016.

39. See Paul Ramsey, *Patient as Person* (New Haven: Yale University Press, 1970), 113–64; Arthur Dyck, "An Alternative to the Ethic of Euthanasia," in R. M. Williams, ed., *To Live and To Die: When Why and How* (New York: Springer Verlag, 1973), 98–112.

40. *In re Quinlan* 355 A.2d 647 (1976).

41. Veatch, *Death, Dying and the Biological Revolution,* 197–200; Germain Grisez and Joseph Boyle, *Life and Death with Liberty and Justice* (South Bend, Ind.: University of Notre Dame Press, 1978), 86–120. Also see the various right-to-die court cases, in which courts routinely fall back on this kind of framework.

42. Two versions of this position can be seen in James Childress, *Who Decides* (New York: Oxford University Press, 1983); Charles Culver and Bernard Gert, *Philosophy of Medicine: Conceptual and Ethical Issues in Medicine and Psychiatry* (New York: Oxford University Press, 1982).

43. I have worked this out in some more detail in a forthcoming paper, "Competency and Social Rationality," *Journal of Medicine and Philosophy.* Also we might note that in practice competency assessments are quite frequently rooted in a socially contingent judgment about the plausibility of what it is that the agent proposes to do. See Eric Cassel, "What is the Aim of Medicine," *Death and Decision,* ed. Ernan McMullin, (Greeley, Colorado: Westview Press, 1978), 13–27.

44. H. T. Englehardt, "Medicine and the Concept of a Person," in T. Beauchamp, ed. *Ethical Issues in Death and Dying,* (Englewood Cliffs: Prentice, 1978); Michael Tooley, "A Defense of Abortion and Infanticide," in *The Problem of Abortion,* ed. Joel Feinberg (Belmont, California: Wadsworth, 1973), 51–91.

45. Englehardt, "Medicine and the Concept of a Person"; H. T. Engelhardt, "Defining Death: A Problem for Law and Medicine," *Annals of Respiratory Diseases* 112 (1975): 587; Robert Veatch, "The Whole Brain Oriented Concept of Death: An Outmoded Philosophical Formulation," *Journal of Thanatology* 3 (1975): 13–30.

46. See Julius Korein, "The Problem of Brain Death," *Annals of the New York Academy of Science* 315 (1978): 19–38; Grisez and Boyle, *Life and Death with Liberty and Justice,* 59–61; James Bernat, Charles Culver and Bernard Gert, "On the Definition and Criterion of Death," *Annals of Internal Medicine* 94 (1981): 389–94; President's Commission for the Study of Ethical Problems in Medicine and Biomedical and Behavioral Research, *Defining Death* (Washington, D.C.: US Government Printing Office, 1981).

47. Englehardt, "Medicine and the Concept of a Person," 272–73.

48. Carson Strong, "Positive Killing and the Permanently Unconscious Patient," *Bioethics Quarterly* 3 (1981): 190–205.

286

49. Englehardt, "Medicine and the Concept of a Person."

50. Arval Morris, "Law, Morality and Euthanasia for the Severely Defective Newborn," in M. Kohl, ed., *Infanticide and the Value of Life* (Buffalo: Prometheus Books, 1979), 137–58; Arval Morris, "Voluntary Euthanasia," *Washington Law Review* 45 (1970): 239–71.

51. Morris, "Voluntary Euthanasia," 267.

52. See especially Diana Crane, *The Sanctity of Social Life* (New York: Russel Sage, 1976). Crane found a very wide disparity among physicians in judgments on withdrawing or withholding therapy. Her work is discussed in more detail in chapter seven. Also see Joy Skeel and Ron Benson, "Medical Indications for Postponing Death," paper delivered at meeting of the American Academy of Religion, at New Orleans, La., 1978; and Robert Pearlman et al., "Variability in Physician Bioethical Decisionmaking: A Case Study of Euthanasia," *Annals of Internal Medicine* 97 (1982): 420–25.

53. See Mannes, *Last Rights*; Daniel McGuire, *Death by Choice* (New York: Schocken Books, 1973).

54. Ellen Suckiel, "Death and Benefit in the Permanently Unconscious Patient," *Journal of Medicine and Philosophy* 3 (1978): 38–52.

55. W. Steele and J. Hill, "A Plea for the Legal Right to Die," *Oklahoma Law Review* 29 (1976): 328–48; Richard Delgado, "Euthanasia Reconsidered," *Arizona Law Review* 17 (1975): 826–56; Morris Forkosch, "Privacy, Human Dignity and Euthanasia: Are These Independent Constitutional Rights?" *University of San Fernando Valley Law Review* 3 (1974): 1–25.

56. Veatch, *Death, Dying and the Biological Revolution*, 110–15; Benedict Ashley and Kevin O'Rourke, *Health Care Ethics* (St. Louis: Catholic Hospital Association, 1982), 381–88; E. W. Kluge, *The Ethics of Deliberate Death* (Port Washington, N.Y.: Kennikat Press, 1981).

57. The essential text in presenting the case for mercy killing and assisted suicide is Derek Humphry, *Let Me Die Before I Wake* (New York: Hemlock Society, 1985).

58. The cases are too numerous to cite in any detail. We can note two recent cases, however, as instances of the widely disparate treatment of these sorts of cases in law. In Florida, Roswell Gilbert was sentenced to life in prison for the murder of his sixty-two-year-old wife, who suffered from Alzheimer's disease and begged to be killed. His appeals were rejected by the courts and by the Florida Board of Pardons; see *New York Times* August 21, August 28, 1985. At the same

time in New York, Kurt Semel was not charged for the suffocation of his terminally ill wife when she had also begged to be killed. See *New York Times* August 13, 1985.

59. *In re Quinlan*, 355 A.2d 647.

60. See above, 138–39.

61. *In re Quinlan*, 661–62.

62. *In re Quinlan*, 661–62.

63. *John F. Kennedy Memorial Hospital* v. *Heston* 179 A. 2d. 670 (1976).

64. *In re Quinlan* 355 A. 2d 661–62.

65. *In re Quinlan* at 663.

66. *Superintendent of Belchertown State Hospital* v. *Saikewicz* 370 N.E. 2d 417 (1976); *In re Spring* 405 N.E. 2d 115 (1980).

67. *Superintendent of Belchertown State Hospital* v. *Saikewicz* 370 N.E. 2d 417 (1976), at 430.

68. *Superintendent of Belchertown State Hospital* v. *Saikewicz* 370 N.E. 2d 417 (1976), at 430.

69. *In re Spring* 405 N.E. 2d 115 (1980).

70. *In re Spring* 405 N.E. 2d 115 (1980), at 120.

71. This point has been noted even by those sympathetic to the result achieved. See George Annas, "Quality of Life in the Courts, *Hastings Center Reports* 8 (August 1980): 9–10.

72. *In re* Application of Eichner 423 N.Y.S. 2d 580 (1979), at 591 Affd. *sub nom Eichner* v. *Dillon* 426 N.Y.S. 2d 517.

73. *In re* Application of Eichner 423 N.Y.S. 2d 580 (1979), at 591 Affd. *sub nom Eichner* v. *Dillon* 426 N.Y.S. 2d 517 at 584.

74. *In re* Application of Eichner 423 N.Y.S. 2d 580 (1979), at 591 Affd. *sub nom Eichner* v. *Dillon* 426 N.Y.S. 2d 517 at 593.

75. 426 N.Y.S. 2d at 536.

76. 426 N.Y.S. 2d at 545.

77. 426 N.Y.S. 2d at 545.

78. *In re Storar* 52 N.Y. 2d 363.

79. The AMA stand has just been approved by its nine member judicial council. Though it does not represent the opinion of all physicians, it is an authoritative decision of the professional association. See *New York Times*, March 18, 1986.

80. For the *Herbert* case, see especially *Los Angeles Times,* May 5, 1983, and Bonnie Steinbock, "The Removal of Mr. Herbert's Feeding Tube," *Hastings Center Report* 13 (October 1983):13–16.

81. For details of the *Conroy* case, see Richard McCormick, "Caring or Starving? The Case of Claire Conroy," *America* (April 6, 1985): 269–73; also *Matter of Conroy* 486 A2d 1209.

82. For the debate, see Joanne Lynn and James Childress, "Must Patients Always be Given Food and Water?" *Hastings Center Report* 13 (October 1983): 17–24; Gilbert Meilander, "On Removing Food and Water," *Hastings Center Report* 14 (December 1984): 11–I3; K. C. Micetich, P. Steinecker, and D. Thomasma, "Are Intravenous Fluids Morally Required for a Dying Patient?" *Annals of Internal Medicine* 143 (1983): 975–78; Mark Seigler and Alan Weisbard, "Against the Emerging Stream: Should Fluids and Nutritional Support be Discontinued?" *Annals of Internal Medicine* 145 (1985): 129–31; Robert Barry, O.P., "Are Food and Fluids Always Required?" *Journal of Family Studies* 3 (1984): 21–29.

83. See especially Barry, O.P., "Are Food and Fluids Always Required?"; Seigler and Weisbard, "Against the Emerging Stream"; and Meilander, "On Removing Food and Water."

84. *Matter of Conroy* 486 A2d 1209.

85. *Matter of Conroy,* 1221–23.

86. *Matter of Conroy,* 1229–32.

87. *Matter of Conroy,* 1332–35.

88. This point is recognized in the perceptive commentary on *Conroy* by Norman Cantor, "Conroy, Best Interests and the Handling of Dying Patients," *Rutgers Law Review* 37 (1985): 543–77.

89. See below, 259–62.

Chapter Five: *Suicide*

1. Albert Camus, *The Myth of Sysiphus,* trans. J. O'Brien (New York: Vintage Books, 1955).

2. See especially A. Alvarez, *The Savage God* (London: Wiedenfield and Nicholson, 1971); G. Rosen, "History," in S. Perlin, ed., *Handbook for the Study of Suicide* (London: Oxford University Press, 1975), 3–29; Lester Crocker, "The Discussion of Suicide in the Eighteenth Century," *Journal of the History of Ideas* 13 (1952): 47–52; S. E. Sprott, *The*

English Debate on Suicide: From Donne to Hume (Lasalle: Open Court, 1961).

3. The literature here is too vast to even note; for a comprehensive review of the psychological dimensions, see Robert Litman, Norman Faberow and Edwin Schneidman, *The Psychology of Suicide* (New York: Science House, 1970).

4. David Hume, "On Suicide," *Essays: Moral, Political and Literary* (London: Oxford University Press, 1963), 585–96. On Hume, see also Tom Beauchamp, "Analysis of Hume's Essay on Suicide," *Review of Metaphysics* 30 (1976): 71–95. See also Baron Montesquieu, *Persian Letters*, no. 76; John Donne, *Biothánatos* (London, 1646; New York: Facsimile Text Society, 1930); Rousseau, *Julie ou la Nouvelle Heloise*, part 3, letters 21 and 22; Nietzsche, *Thus Spake Zarathustra*, part 1, section 21.

5. Aside from Hume and Nietzsche, the most trenchant presentation of this position at present is by Thomas Szaz. See Thomas Szaz, "The Ethics of Suicide" *Antioch Review* 3 (Spring 1971): 7–17; see also A. Kobler, "Suicide: Right and Reason," *Bioethics Quarterly* 2 (1980): 46–55; Eliot Slater, "Choosing the Time to Die," in M. P. Battin and D. Mayo, eds., *Suicide: The Philosophical Issues* (New York: Macmillan, 1980), 200–206.

6. Hume, "On Suicide," 585–86.

7. Szaz, "Ethics of Suicide," 13.

8. Slater, "Choosing the Time to Die," 202.

9. In this respect the criticism of modern ethical theory by Alastair Macintyre and Stanley Hauerwas is correct; Macintyre especially is on target when he argues that Nietzsche reveals the essence of modernity in this regard. See Alastair Macintyre, *After Virtue* (South Bend: Notre Dame, 1979).

10. David Greenburg, "Involuntary Psychiatric Commitments to Prevent Suicide," *New York University Law Review* 49 (1974): 227–69. In the same vein but more nuanced in sociology, see Jack Douglas, *The Social Meaning of Suicide* (Princeton: Princeton University Press, 1967).

11. In both Hobbes and Locke, the state of nature is a state of perpetual war of all against all. It is precisely in order not to live as natural men that human beings form a political regime. See Hobbes, *Leviathan* 2:17–18; Locke, *Two Treatises* 2:9–10.

12. For an example of this move, see H. B. Brandt, "The Morality

and Rationality of Suicide," in Perlin, ed., *Handbook for the Study of Suicide*, 61–76.

13. Bruce Ennis and Richard Emery, *The Rights of Mental Patients* (New York: Avon Books, 1978), 49.

14. R. Barraclough et al., "A Hundred Cases of Suicide: Clinical Aspects," *British Journal of Psychiatry* 125 (1974): 355–73.

15. For a comprehensive review of the literature plus a replication of the British results, see Jan Beskow, *Suicide and Mental Disorder in Swedish Men, Acta Psychiatrica Scandinavica*, supp. 277 (1979); D. Lester, "The Relationship of Mental Disorder to Suicidal Behavior," *New York State Journal of Medicine* 71 (1971): 1503–5.

16. Rolf Sartorius, "Paternalistic Grounds for Involuntary Civil Commitment: A Utilitarian Perspective," in Tristram Englehardt and Baruch Brody, eds., *Mental Illness: Law and Public Policy* (Boston: D. Reidel, 1980), 144.

17. See especially Paul Applebaum et al., "Empirical Assessment of Competency to Consent to Psychiatric Care," *American Journal of Psychiatry* 138 (1981): 1170–76; A. Lewis, "Melancholia: A Clinical Survey of Depressed States," *Journal of Medical Science* 80 (1934): 277–378; E. Kraepelin, *Manic Depressive Illness and Paranoia* (Edinburgh: E. and S. Livingstone, 1924); R. M. Cohen et al., "Effort and Cognition in Depression," *Archives of General Psychiatry* 39 (1982): 593–97.

18. Ennis and Emery, *Rights of Mental Patients*.

19. The classic essay on this is A. Rosen, "Detection of Suicidal Patients: An Example of Some Limitations on the Prediction of Infrequent Events," *Journal of Consulting Psychology* 18 (1954): 397–403; see also D. Lester, "Attempts to Predict Suicidal Risk Using Psychological Tests," *Psychiatry Bulletin* 74 (1970): 1–17; G. Murphy, "Clinical Identification of Suicide Risk," *Archives of General Psychiatry* 27 (1972): 356–60.

20. C. Bagely and S. Greer, "The Effectiveness of Psychiatry Intervention in Attempted Suicide," *British Medical Journal* 1 (1971): 310–12; C. Bagely, "The Evaluation of a Suicide Prevention Scheme by an Ecological Method," *Sociological Science and Medicine* 2 (1968): 1–4; Robert Litman, "Beyond Crisis," in Edwin Schneidman, ed., *Suicidology: Contemporary Developments* (New York: Grune and Stratton, 1976).

21. John Locke, *Second Treatise of Government*, c. 2, paragraphs 1–6.

22. Gary Glenn, "Inalienable Rights and Positive Government in the Modern World," *Journal of Politics* 41 (1979): 1056–80; Gary Glenn, "Inalienable Rights and Locke's Argument for Limited Government: Political Implications of a Right to Suicide," *Journal of Politics* 46 (1984): 81–105. The question of *inalienable rights* was of central importance in the emergence of liberal theory; for an overview—with which I do not entirely agree—see R. Tuck, *Natural Rights: Their Origin and Development* (New York: Cambridge University Press, 1979).

23. Locke, *Second Treatise of Government*, c. 2, par. 6; see George Windstrup, "Locke on Suicide," *Political Theory* 8 (1980): 169–82.

24. John Locke, *An Essay Concerning Human Understanding*, Book 4, c. 10.

25. John Locke, *The Reasonableness of Christianity*; on the political nature of Locke's religious teaching, see W. Blum, N. Wintfield, S. Teger, "Locke's Idea of God: Rational Truth or Political Myth," *Journal of Politics* 42 (1980): 416–38.

26. See above, 71–73.

27. Locke, *Second Treatise*, c. 2, par. 6.

28. Plato, *Phaedo*, 61c–62d.

29. Plato, *Phaedo*, 61c–62d.

30. Plato, *Laws*, 873 ff.

31. Plato, *Apology*, 27b–28c; *Phaedo*, 61d.

32. See Greenburgh "Involuntary Psychiatric Commitments to Prevent Suicide"; Germain Grisez and Joseph Boyle, *Life and Death with Liberty and Justice* (South Bend: Notre Dame University Press, 1979), 121–38; Karen Lebacqz and Tristram Englehardt, "Suicide," in Dennis Horan and David Mall, eds., *Death, Dying and Euthanasia* (Fredricksburg, Md.: University Publications of America, 1977), 669–705.

33. Karen Lebacqz and Tristram Englehardt, "Suicide," 669. See Anthony Flew, "The Principle of Euthanasia," in A. B. Downing, ed., *Euthanasia and the Right to Die* (London: Peter Owen, 1969), 17.

34. Leslie Francis, "Assisting Suicide: A Problem for the Criminal Law," in Battin and Mayo, eds., *Suicide: The Philosophical Issues*, 263–64.

35. Lebacqz and Englehardt, "Suicide," 690–91.

36. Lebacqz and Englehardt, "Suicide," 690.

37. Francis, "Assisting Suicide," 263.

38. Lebacqz and Englehardt, "Suicide," 692.

39. Alan Sullivan, "A Constitutional Right to Suicide?" in Battin and Mayo, eds., *Suicide: The Philosophical Issues*, 244.

40. See the discussion of these competency issues in chapter seven.

41. M. P. Battin, "Manipulated Suicide," *Bioethics Quarterly* 2 (1980): 123–34.

42. Greenburgh, "Involuntary Psychiatric Commitments to Prevent Suicide," 232–33; Grisez and Boyle, *Life and Death with Liberty and Justice*, 229–30.

43. Erwin Stengel, *Suicide and Attempted Suicide* (New York: Jason Aronson, 1974).

Chapter Six: *Abortion*

1. See Alexander Bickel, *The Least Dangerous Branch* (New York: 1962); John Hart Ely, *Democracy and Distrust* (Cambridge: Harvard University Press, 1980).

2. *Roe* v. *Wade* 410 U.S. 116 at 135.

3. *Roe* v. *Wade* 410 U.S. 116 at 130

4. See Philip Haymann and Douglas Barzelay, "The Forest and the Trees: *Roe* v. *Wade* and Its Critics," *Boston University Law Review* 63 (1973): 765, 769. Laurence Tribe, "Forward to the Supreme Court— 1972 Term: Toward a Model of Roles in the Due Process of Life and Law," *Harvard Law Review* 87 (1973): 20–23. Laurence Tribe, *American Constitutional Law* (Mineola, N.Y.: Foundation Press, 1978), 928 ff.; Michael Perry, "Abortion, Public Morals and the Police Power: The Ethical Function of Substantive Due Process," *UCLA. Law Review* 23 (1976): 689–736; Donald Regan, "Rewriting *Roe* v. *Wade*," in Vinoviskis and Carl Schneider, eds., *The Law and Politics* of Abortion (Lexington: D. C. Heath, 1980), 3–80.

5. See Karen Lebacqz, "Prenatal Diagnosis and Selective Abortion," *Linacre Quarterly* 40 (1973): 109–27.

6. Any good textbook in embryology will review the essential facts at this point; a good brief review is contained in Bart Heffernan, M.D. "The Early Biography of Everyman," in Thomas Hilgers and Dennis Horan, eds., *Abortion and Social Justice* (New York: Sheed and Ward, 1972), 3–25.

7. Selective abortion cannot possibly be performed before nine-teen–twenty-one weeks gestational age, at which point the fetus simply cannot be distinguished from the newborn infant in any relevant way. See my essay, "The Moral Quandary of Pre-Natal Genetics," in press.

8. The most important version of this position is that provided by Michael Tooley, "Abortion and Infanticide," *Philosophy and Public Affairs* 2 (1972): 37–65. Tooley is quite open in his defense of infanticide, but he attempts to avoid the broader implications noted in the text by simply postulating various versions of his central thesis such that abortion is permitted and involuntary euthanasia of all incompetent persons is not. None of these moves is cogent. See Gary Jones, "Rights and Desires," *Ethics* 92 (1981): 52–56.

9. Laurence Becker, "Human Being: the Boundaries of the Concept," *Philosophy and Public Affairs* 4: (1975): 334–59.

10. Becker, "Human Being," 336.

11. Becker, "Human Being," 337.

12. Becker, "Human Being," 344–45.

13. For a most cogent attempt to argue that human life and its attendant moral status must be said to begin at conception, see Richard Werner, "Abortion: The Moral Status of the Unborn," *Social Theory and Practice* 3 (1974): 201–22. The view I have developed in this chapter is similar to that developed by Baruch Brody, *Abortion and the Sanctity of Human Life: A Philosophical View,* (Cambridge: MIT Press, 1975).

14. This view is found in many popular defenses of abortion on demand, but the most prestigious presentation is that found in John Peel, Malcolm Potts, and Peter Diggory, *Abortion.* (New York: Cambridge University Press, 1977), 132–53.

15. I have reviewed these data in "The Demographic Argument for Liberal Abortion Policies: Analysis of a Pseudo Issue," *New Perspectives on Human Abortion,* eds. Thomas Hilgers, Dennis Horan, and David Mall (Fredericks, Md.: University Press of America, 1981), 450–65.

16. For example, Mehlan found that a decade after the liberalization of abortion law in Roumania, women seeking abortion at the largest women's hospital in Bucharest had an average of 3.9 previous abortions. So high a figure is demographically impossible unless these women were using abortion as a primary means of contracep-

tion. K. H. Mehlan, "Legal Abortions in Roumania," *Journal of Sex Research* 1 (1965): 31–38; for the same phenomenon in America, see Kristin Luker, *Taking Chances: Abortion and the Decision not to Contracept* (Berkeley: University of California Press, 1978).

17. C. B. Goodhart, "Estimation of Illegal Abortions," *Journal of Biosocial Science* 1 (1969): 235–45.

18. See C. B. Goodhart, "The Frequency of Illegal Abortion," *Eugenics Review* 55 (1964): 197–200.

19. Barbara Syska, Thomas Hilgers, and Dennis O'Hare, "An Objective Model for Estimating Criminal Abortions and its Implications for Public Policy," *New Perspectives*, 164–81.

20. Syska, Hilgers, and O'Hare, "Objective Model for Estimating Criminal Abortions," 178.

21. The earliest and most authoritative statement of this view is in Tribe, "Forward to the Supreme Court—1972 Term." Unlike many other authors, Tribe eventually saw the flaws in this position and abandoned it.

22. See Winthrop Jordan, *White over Black* (Chapel Hill: University of North Carolina Press, 1968); Lewis Hanke *All Mankind is One* (De Kalb, Ill.: Northern Illinois University Press, 1974).

23. Frederick Jaffe, "Enacting Religious Beliefs in a Pluralistic Society," Hastings Center Report 8 (August 1978): 15.

24. Such a position has been argued by many philosophers who have concentrated on what they viewed as a parasitical relationship between the mother and the fetus as well as by legal scholars seeking to defend Roe. The most well-known version is from Judith Jarvis Thompson, "A Defense of Abortion," *Philosophy and Public Affairs* 1 (1971): 47–66. From the legal field, the most trenchant version is found in Regan, "Rewriting *Roe v. Wade*."

25. Regan, "Rewriting *Roe v. Wade*," 7–13.

26. S. 158 98th Congress, 1st session.

27. Senate Joint Res. 140 90th Congress 2nd session.

28. The most cogent presentation of this view is in John Noonan, *A Private Choice* (New York: Free Press, 1979), 180–85.

29. Germain Grisez and Joseph Boyle, *Life and Death with Liberty and Justice* (South Bend: University of Notre Dame Press, 1979), 309–10 contains an example of such an unwieldy amendment that attempts to cover every contingency.

30. See Charles McIlwain, *Constitutionalism* (Ithaca: Cornell University Press, 1948) and Joseph Cropsey, "The United States as a Regime and the Sources of the American Way of Life," in Robert Horwitz, ed., *The Moral Foundation of the American Republic* (Charlottesville: University of Virginia Press, 1977), 86–107; Aristotle says, "A constitution may be defined as an organization of offices in a state by which the method of their distribution is fixed, the sovereign authority is determined and the nature of the end to be pursued by the association and all its members is prescribed. Laws, as distinct from the frame of the constitution are rules by which the magistrates should exercise their powers and should watch and check transgressors. It follows . . . that we must always bear in mind the varieties of each constitution and the number of those varieties in order to be able to enact laws appropriate to each. *Politics* 1289a.

31. Generally what law existed was common, rather than statutory, law. The latter did not come until the nineteenth century. See generally Robert Destro, "Abortion and the Constitution," *California Law Review* 63 (1975): 1250–351, especially 1267–73; James Mohr, *Abortion in America: The Origins and Evolution of a National Policy* (New York: Oxford University Press, 1978). For the common law at the time of the founding, see Blackstone, *Commentary on the Laws of England* 4:394–95.

32. Aristotle, *History of Animals*, 583b; For a review of some of the ways this view was worked out morally, see John Noonan, Jr., "An Almost Absolute Value in History," in Noonan, ed., *The Morality of Abortion* (Cambridge: Harvard University Press, 1970), 1–59.

33. The best example is the duty to retreat in the face of an attack by someone using deadly force. "The courts . . . differ to such an extent upon the question of the necessity of retreating before an assailant in order to justify a killing in self defense that doubts have been expressed as to what is the prevailing doctrine." 40 Jur. Am. 2d 449–56. In some jurisdictions, one could be charged with second degree murder for an act that in other states would be classed as self-defense.

34. For a useful review of federalism, see William Ebenstein et al., *American Democracy* (New York: Harper and Row, 1967), 158–83; also see the important collection of essays edited by Robert Goldwin, *A Nation of States: Essays on the American Federal System* (Chicago: Rand McNally, 1974).

35. Charles Rice, *In the Name of Freedom* (Chicago: Franciscan Herald Press, 1977), 123.

36. The most telling example here, aside from the case of prohibition, is the repeated, nearly successful attempts, to amend the constitution to provide for prayer in public schools, although many Catholic and Jewish parents are deeply suspicious of such efforts, let alone those parents who profess no religious faith whatsoever. Also we may note the building majority that seeks serious restrictions on the dissemination of pornographic materials, especially via electronic media.

37. The original Hatch proposal was eventually amended to include only section one. Although the original was a sounder proposal, even the amended proposal failed in congress. The amended version was, however, still a superior resolution to the abortion controversy over all other proposals.

Chapter Seven: *From Policy to Practice*

1. See I. Jenkins, *Social Order and the Limits of Law* (Princeton: Princeton University Press, 1980) for an excellent statement on the limitations of law and policy as guides of human action.

2. Paul Ramsey, *The Patient as Person* (New Haven: Yale University Press, 1970), 113–64.

3. See below, 238.

4. Diana Crane, *The Sanctity of Social Life* (New York: Russel Sage, 1976).

5. Crane, *Sanctity of Social Life*, 40–46.

6. Crane, *Sanctity of Social Life*, 35–40.

7. Crane, *Sanctity of Social Life*, 49–52; see also cases a1 and a2, 227.

8. Crane, *Sanctity of Social Life*, 221.

9. Crane, *Sanctity of Social Life*, 229–30.

10. Crane, *Sanctity of Social Life*, 258, case b3.

11. Robert Pearlmen et al., "Variability in Physician Bioethical Decisionmaking," *Annals of Internal Medicine* 97 (1982): 420–25.

12. N. K. Brown and D. J. Thompson, "Non-Treatment of Fever in Extended Care Facilities," *New England Journal of Medicine* 300 (1979): 1246–50.

13. Raymond Duff and A. G. M. Campbell, "Moral and Ethical Dilemmas in the Special Care Nursery," *New England Journal of Medicine* 289 (1973): 890–94.

14. Duff and Campbell, "Moral and Ethical Dilemmas," 892.

15. Raymond Duff, "On Deciding the Care of Defective Infants," in Marvin Kohl, ed., *Infanticide and the Value of Life* (Buffalo: Prometheus Books, 1979), 96–101.

16. S. J. Youngner et al., "Do Not Resuscitate Orders: Incidence and Implications in a Medical Intensive Care Unit," *Journal of the American Medical Association* 253 (1985): 54–57.

17. These are compiled in an appendix to the report of the President's Commission for the Study of Ethical Problems in Medicine and Bio-medical and Behavioral Research, *Deciding to Forgo Life-Sustaining Treatment* (Washington, D. C.: US Government Printing Office), 494–545.

18. See for example the guidelines from the New York and Minnesota medical societies, and Beth Israel Hospital in Boston, all in the appendix to the Report of the President's Commission.

19. Report of the President's Commission, 510–16. I would also call attention to the fact that all but one of the state "living will" statutes limits the operation of the law to terminally ill patients. In other words, only when the patient is terminally ill may or must—it varies in the statutes—a physician honor the patient's written request for no further treatment.

20. This point about the priority of "vision" or description in evaluation can be made in several ways, and has been advanced by a number of important contemporary theories. For the best examples, see Stanley Hauerwas, *Vision and Virtue* (South Bend: Notre Dame University Press, 1974), especially 1–90; Stanley Hauerwas, *Truthfulness and Tragedy* (South Bend: Notre Dame University Press, 1977); Eric D'Arcy, *Human Acts: an Essay in Their Moral Evaluation* (Oxford: Clarendon Press, 1963).

21. See Paul Ramsey, *Ethics at the Edges of Life* (New Haven: Yale University Press, 1979), 160–71; R. B. Zachary, "The Neonatal Surgeon," *British Medical Journal* 2 (October 9, 1976): 866–69; R. B. Zachary, "Ethical and Social Aspects of Treatment for Spina Bifida," *Lancet* 2 (1968): 274–77.

22. See above, 151–68.

23. See H. L. A. Hart, *The Concept of Law* (Oxford: Clarendon Press, 1961), 77–96. This point about the open texture of specific legal or moral rules is meant to apply only to *specific* rules, or what an older

terminology would have called the "secondary precepts" of the natural law. Hart terms them secondary rules, while Ramsey calls them rules as distinct from general principles. While admitting that such legal rules must have an open texture, I do not admit that there are no exceptionless principles in Ramsey's terminology. Considerations advanced by Ramsey and Dworkin among others seem to me to decisively point toward such principles, at least in our political and legal tradition. For example, it seems to me that the principle of equal treatment under law, or the equal worth of individual lives is such a principle. In fact, it is precisely our adherence to such principles that makes the whole notion of exceptions intelligible. For the need to show that a given case is an exception only follows if, *prima facie*, a rule that seems to apply to this case generates a different conclusion. But if we did not accept the equal applicability of rules, then the need to create an exception would vanish. See Paul Ramsey, "The Case of the Curious Exception," in *Norm and Context in Christian Ethics*, Paul Ramsey and Gene Outka, eds. (New York: Charles Scribners, 1968), 67–135; Leonard Miller, "Rules and Exceptions," *Ethics* 66 (1956), 272–80.

24. Lon Fuller, *The Morality of Law* (New Haven: Yale University Press, 1964), 33–94, 159–62.

25. I disagree almost entirely with Dworkin's conclusions on particular cases, and with much of his defense of judicial discretion; yet I think that his defense of the concept of rights and their importance in the adjudication of cases at law does reflect something very important about our political and legal tradition. This is especially true of his analysis of the place of general principles in adjudication, principles that are not found stated in specific statutory language but are nonetheless crucial in understanding our legal and political tradition. See Ronald Dworkin, *Taking Rights Seriously* (Cambridge: Harvard University Press, 1977.)

26. See above, 193–94.

27. See above, 131–36.

28. Some theorists have argued that a "right to do wrong" is impossible. See William Godwin, *Enquiry Concerning Political Justice*, ed. K. C. Carter (Oxford: Clarendon Press, 1971), 88; John Mackie, "Can There Be a Right-Based Moral Theory?" *Midwest Studies in Philosophy* 3 (1978), 350–59; for a response that still proves my point, see Jeremy Waldron, "A Right to Do Wrong," *Ethics* 92 (1981), 21–39. The relationship between rights and right is important and has been ex-

plored by several contemporary theorists with various degrees of cogency. I cannot develop the matter further here, but for an excellent entré to the issue, one can consult John Finnie, *Natural Law and Natural Rights* (Oxford: Clarendon Press, 1981); also see Lisa Cahill, "Toward a Christian Theory of Human Rights," *Journal of Religious Ethics* 8 (1981), 281–301.

29. See Dworkin, *Taking Rights Seriously,* 260–68; James Childress, *Who Should Decide: Paternalism in Health Care* (New York: Oxford University Press, 1982), 67–69.

30. At times even Childress seems to admit such a prudential basis for many liberty rights. See Childress, *Who Should Decide,* 69.

31. See 198.

32. Sometimes, however, the results of nonintervention are so patently untenable that even very strenuous acts are justified, such as someone forcibly preventing a stranger from jumping off a building. This issue has been raised recently by cases in which courts have ordered women to have caesarian sections that were believed to be necessary to save the life of the baby when to do so would require the use of blood transfusions or in other ways violate their religious beliefs. In the leading such case, the court concluded correctly that the value of innocent human life is paramount in such a case and ordered the surgery. *Jefferson v. Griffin Spaulding County Hospital Authority* 247 S.E. 2d 457 (1981).

33. I would point out here that, unlike some questions, such as the case of the permanently comatose patient, there has never been a broad social consensus on the question of abortion on demand. There are sharp divisions on the question as there have been for a decade, but substantial pluralities can be found on all sides of the question. Therefore, purely as a matter of policy, a rejection of current practice would be no more controversial or without support than was *Roe.*

34. The relevant material on the procedure is found in Jack A. Pritchard and Paul C. MacDonald, *Williams Obstetrics,* 16th ed. (New York: Appleton-Century Crofts, 1980), 330–40.

35. See above, 110.

36. On Down's syndrome see H. Robinson and N. Robinson, *The Mentally Retarded Child* (New York: McGraw Hill, 1976).

37. See generally AMA Council of Scientific Affairs, "Maternal Serum A-Fetoprotein Monitoring," *Journal of the American Medical Association* 247 (1982): 1478–82; G. B. Kolata, "Mass Screening for Neu-

ral Tube Defects," *Hastings Center Report* 10 (December 1980): 8–10; Pritchard and MacDonald, *Williams Obstetrics,* 339–44. Even the diagnosis of the open lesion and its location on the spinal column—a crucial element in prognosis—is very difficult *in utero.* See especially J. C. Hobbins et al., "Stage II Ultrasound Examination for the Diagnosis of Fetal Abnormalities with an Elevated Amniotic Fluid A-Fetoprotein Concentration," *American Journal of Obstetrics and Gynecology* 142 (1982): 1026–29; H. P. Robinson, "Detection of Birth Defects by Ultrasonography," *Birth Defects* 17 (1981): 17–30.

38. John Lorber, "Result of Treatment of Myelomeningocele," *Developmental Medicine and Child Neurology* 13 (1971): 279–33. The literature on this subject is vast, but the best newer studies support two points: 1) even in the worst prognostic category, the majority of children will eventually have IQs in the normal, borderline, or mildly retarded range, surely not such outcomes that could even plausibly be said to be a life not worth living; and 2) in the vast majority of cases, the eventual quality of life of the child cannot be known very well at all at birth. See A. Soare and P. Raimondi, "Intellectual and Perceptual Motor Characteristics of Treated Myelomeningocele Children," *American Journal of Diseases of Children* 131 (1977): 199–206; J. T. Brown and D. G. McLone, "Treatment Choices for the Infant with Myelomeningocele," in Dennis Horan and Melinda Delhoyde, eds., *Infanticide and the Handicapped Newborn* (Provo: Brigham Young University Press, 1981), 69–75. From these studies the interested reader can find ample sources to pursue this matter further.

39. The most interesting example in this regard was the statement of the Roman Catholic Bishop of New Jersey, the religious superior of the Quinlans' own pastor. See Bishop Lawrence Casey, "A Statement on the Case of Karen Quinlan," *Catholic Mind* 74 (1976): 12–18.

40. See A. Crenvik et al., "Cessation of Therapy in Terminal Illness," *Critical Care Medicine* 6 (1978): 284–88; David Levy et al., "Prognosis in Non-Traumatic Coma," *Annals of Internal Medicine* 94 (1981): 293–97; James Heiden et al., "Severe Head Injury and Outcome," in A. J. Popp, ed., *Neural Trauma* (New York: Raven Press, 1979), 327–40. These various studies are confirmed in the Report of the President's Commission, *Defining Death,* 90–100. The commission's own study at four hospitals confirmed the very grim prognosis for survival of those who remained comatose at one month after the onset of coma.

41. This point is controversial and I state it here as one tentative

way in which these cases may be handled. If sound, it would provide a justification for removing life supporting care from Karen Quinlan, but not from Claire Conroy who was sentient—that is, aware of being alive.

42. I have worked out some of these ideas in a paper delivered at the National Conference on Handicapped Newborns, Fordham University, March, 1985, "Babies Doe: The Moral Basis of a Policy Consensus." The papers from the conference will appear in James Bopp and Richard Sherlock, eds., *Handicapped Newborns in American Society* (Frederick, Md.: University Publications of America, 1986). Also see Carson Strong, "Positive Killing and the Permanently Unconscious Patient," *Bioethics Quarterly* 3 (1981): 190–205; Joel Feinberg, "The Rights of Animals and Unborn Generations" in W. Blackstone, ed., *Philosophy and the Environmental Crisis* (Athens: University of Georgia Press, 1974), 189–211.

43. Paul Ramsey, *The Patient as Person* (New Haven: Yale University Press, 1970).

Conclusion

1. Dietrich Bonhoeffer, *Ethics*, ed. E. Bethge (New York: Macmillan Co., 1969), 163–64.

2. Sebastian de Grazia, *The Political Community* (Chicago: University of Chicago Press, 1949), 3.

3. Roscoe Pound, "Justice According to Law," *Columbia Law Review* 13 (1913): 706.

Bibliography

AMA Council of Scientific Affairs. "Maternal Serum A-Fetoprotein Monitoring," *Journal of the American Medical Association*
247 (1982): 1478–82.

Aaron, H. J., and W. B. Schwartz. *The Painful Prescription.*
Washington, D.C.: Brookings Institution, 1984.

Ackerman, Terrence. "Myelomeningocele and Parental Commitment: A Policy Proposal Regarding Selection for Treatment." *Man and Medicine* 5 (1980): 291–303.

Al-Farabi. *The Political Regime.* in M. Mahdi and R. Lerner, ed.
Medieval Political Philosophy. New York: The Free Press,
1962, 31–57.

_____. *The Attainment of Happiness.* in M. Mahdi and R. Lerner,
ed. *Medieval Political Philosophy.* New York: The Free Press,
1962, 57–82.

Alvarez, A. *The Savage God.* London: Wiedenfield and Nicholson, 1971.

Amundsen, D. "The Physician's Obligation to Prolong Life: A
Medical Duty without Classical Roots." *Hastings Center Report* 8 (1978): 23–30.

303

Anderson, J. G. "Demographic Factors Affecting Health Services Utilization." *Medical Care* 11 (1973): 104–20.

Angell, M. "Handicapped Children: Uncle Sam and Baby Doe." *New England Journal of Medicine* 309 (1983): 659–61.

Annas, George. "Quality of Life in the Courts." *Hastings Center Reports* 8 (August 1980): 9–10.

_____. "When Suicide Prevention Becomes Brutality." *Hastings Center Report* 14 (April 1984): 20–22.

Applebaum, Paul, et al. "Empirical Assessment of Competency to Consent to Psychiatric Care." *American Journal of Psychiatry* 138 (1981): 1170–76.

Aristotle. *History of Animals.* Translated by R. Cresswell. London: G. Bell, 1878.

_____. *The Politics.* Edited and Translated by Ernest Barker. New York: Oxford University Press, 1949.

_____. *The Politics.* Edited by W. L. Newman. Oxford: The Clarendon Press, 1902.

_____. *Nichomachean Ethics.* Translated by J. A. K. Thomson. Baltimore: Penguin Books, 1962.

_____. *Rhetoric.* Translated by J. H. Freese. Cambridge: Harvard University Press, 1939.

Arras, John. "Towards an Ethic of Ambiguity." *Hastings Center Report* 14 (April 1984): 24–33.

Arras, John, and Nancy Rhoden. "Withholding Treatment From Baby Doe." *Millbank Memorial Fund Quarterly* 63 (1985): 18–51.

Ashley, Benedict, and Kevin O'Rourke. *Health Care Ethics.* St. Louis: Catholic Health Association, 1982.

Bagely, C. "The Evaluation of a Suicide Prevention Scheme by an Ecological Method." *Sociological Science and Medicine* 2 (1968): 1–4.

Bagely, C., and S. Greer. "The Effectiveness of Psychiatric Intervention in Attempted Suicide." *British Medical Journal* 1 (1971): 310–12.

Bakan, D. *Disease, Pain and Sacrifice.* Chicago: University of Chicago Press, 1968.

Bannion, Anne, M.D. "The Bloomington Baby." *Human Life Review* 7 (Fall 1982): 3–10.

Barraclough, R., et al. "A Hundred Cases of Suicide: Clinical Aspects." *British Journal of Psychiatry* 125 (1974): 355–73.

Barrus, Roger. "The Mormon Founding of Utah," unpublished Ph. D. dissertation, Harvard University, 1984.

Basler, Roy, ed. *Abraham Lincoln: His Speeches and Writings.* Cleveland: World Publishing Co., 1946.

Battin, M. P. "Manipulated Suicide." *Bioethics Quarterly* 2 (1980): 123–34.

Battin, M. P., and D. Mayo, eds. *Suicide: The Philosophical Issues.* New York: Macmillan, 1980.

Beauchamp, Tom. "Analysis of Hume's Essay on Suicide." *Review of Metaphysics* 30 (1976): 71–95.

_____. "Euthanasia," in T. Regan, ed. *Matters of Life and Death,* 67–108.

_____, ed. *Ethical Issues in Death and Dying.* Englewood Cliffs: Prentice, 1978.

Becker, Laurence. "Human Being: the Boundaries of the Concept." *Philosophy and Public Affairs* 4 (1975): 334–59.

Behlmer, George. "Deadly Motherhood: Infanticide and Medical Opinion in Mid-Victorian England." *Journal of the History of Medicine* 35 (1979): 403–27.

Bernat, James, Charles Culver and Bernard Gert. "On the Definition and Criterion of Death." *Annals of Internal Medicine* 94 (1981): 389–94.

Bersath, C. L. "A Neonatalogist Looks at the Baby Doe Rule." *Pediatrics* 72 (1983): 429–29.

Beskow, Jan. *Suicide and Mental Disorder in Swedish Men. Acta Psychiatrica Scandinavica,* supp. 277 (1979).

Bickel, Alexander. *The Least Dangerous Branch.* New York: Viking Books, 1962.

Blackstone, W. *Commentary on the Laws of England.* Edited by W. G. Hammond. San Francisco: Bancroft and Whithey, 1890.

Blackstone, William. "The Meaning and Character of the Equality Principle." *Ethics* 77 (1967): 239–53.

Blum, W., N. Wintfield and S. Teger. "Locke's Idea of God:

Rational Truth or Political Myth." *Journal of Politics* 42 (1980): 416–38.

Boeyink, D. "Pain and Suffering." *Journal of Religious Ethics* 2 (1974): 85–98.

Bok, Sissela, and John Behenke, ed. *Dilemmas of Euthanasia.* New York: Doubleday Anchor, 1975.

Bonhoeffer, Dietrich. *Ethics.* Edited by E. Bethge. New York: Macmillan Co., 1969.

Boyle, Joseph. "On Killing and Letting Die." *New Scholasticism* 51 (1977): 433–52.

_____. "Toward Understanding the Principle of the Double Effect." *Ethics* 90 (1980): 527–38.

Bracton, Henry de. *On the Laws and Customs of England.* 2 vols. Translated by Samuel E. Thorne. Cambridge: Harvard University Press, 1969.

Brandt, Richard. "Defective Newborns and the Morality of Termination," in Kohl, ed.. *Infanticide,* 46–57.

_____. *Ethical Theory.* Englewood Cliffs: Prentice Hall, 1959.

_____. "The Morality and Rationality of Suicide," in Perlin, ed. *Handbook for the Study of Suicide,* 61–76.

Brody, Baruch. *Abortion and the Sanctity of Human Life: A Philosophical View.* Cambridge: MIT Press, 1975.

Brown, J. T., and D. G. McLone. "Treatment Choices for the Infant with Myelomeningocele," in Dennis Horan and Melinda Delhoyde, eds., *Infanticide and the Handicapped Newborn.* Provo: Brigham Young University Press, 1981.

Brown, N. K., and D. J. Thompson. "Non-Treatment of Fever in Extended Care Facilities." *New England Journal of Medicine* 300 (1979): 1246–50.

Burt, Robert. *Taking Care of Strangers.* New York: Free Press, 1979.

Butler, Alan. "Interview."*Newsday,* 9 November 1983.

Chambers, Marcia. "Baby Doe: Hard Case for Parents and Courts." *New York Times,* 8 January 1984.

Childress, James. *Who Should Decide: Paternalism in Health Care.* New York: Oxford University Press, 1982.

Cohen, R. M., et al. "Effort and Cognition in Depression." *Archives of General Psychiatry* 39 (1982): 593–97.

Committee on Bioethics, American Academy of Pediatrics. "Treatment of Critically Ill Newborns." *Pediatrics* 72 (1983): 565–66.

Connery, John. "An Analysis of the HHS Notice on Treating the Handicapped." *Hospital Progress* 62 (1982): 18–20.

Court of Appeals, Brief for Respondents, Stony Brook Hospital and the State University of New York at Stony Brook

Crane, Diana. *The Sanctity of Social Life*. New York: Russel Sage, 1976.

Crenvik, Ake, et al. "Cessation of Therapy in Terminal Illness," *Critical Care Medicine* 6 (1978): 284–88.

Crocker, Lester. "The Discussion of Suicide in the Eighteenth Century." *Journal of the History of Ideas* 13 (1952): 47–52.

Cropsey, Joseph. "The United States as a Regime and the Sources of the American Way of Life," in Robert Horwitz, ed. *The Moral Foundation of the American Republic*. Charlottesville: University of Virginia Press, 1977, 86–107.

Crystal, Stephen. *America's Old Age Crisis*. New York: Basic Books, 1982.

Culver, Charles, and Bernard Gert. *Philosophy of Medicine: Conceptual and Ethical Issues in Medicine and Psychiatry*. New York: Oxford University Press, 1982.

Curran, William. *Harvard Law Review* 71 (1958): 585–89.

D'Arcy, E. "Congenital Defect: Mothers' Reactions to First Information." *British Medical Journal* 3 (1968): 796–800.

D'Arcy, Eric. *Human Acts: an Essay in Their Moral Evaluation*. Oxford: Clarendon Press, 1963.

Damme, Catherine. "Infanticide: The Worth of an Infant Under Law." *Medical History* 22 (1978): 1–24.

De Grazia, Sebastian. *The Political Community*. Chicago: University of Chicago Press, 1948.

De Tocqueville, Alexis. *Democracy in America*. Translated by George Lawrence. New York: Harper and Row, 1966.

Delgado, Richard. "Euthanasia Reconsidered." *Arizona Law Review* 17 (1975): 826–56.

Destro, Robert. "Abortion and the Constitution." *California Law Review* 63 (1975): 1250–351.

Devine, Philip. *The Ethics of Homicide.* Ithaca: Cornell University Press, 1978.

Donne, John. *Biothanatos.* London, 1646; New York: Facsimile Text Society, 1930.

Donnelly, J. "Review of *The Sanctity of Life and the Criminal Law* by Glanville Williams," *Yale Law Journal* 67 (1958): 753–58.

Douglas, Jack. *The Social Meaning of Suicide.* Princeton: Princeton University Press, 1967.

Downing, A. B., ed. *Euthanasia and the Right to Die.* London: Peter Owen, 1969.

Duff, R. A. "Absolute Principles and Double Effect." *Analysis* 36 (1976): 68–80.

Duff, Raymond. "On Deciding the Care of Defective Infants." in Marvin Kohl, ed. *Infanticide and the Value of Life.* Buffalo: Prometheus Books, 1979, 96–101.

———. "On Deciding the Care of Severely Handicapped or Dying Persons." *Pediatrics* 37 (1976): 487–92.

———. "On Deciding the Use of the Family Commons." *Birth Defects: Original Article Series* 12 (1976): 73–84.

Duff, Raymond, and A. G. M. Campbell. "Authors' Response." *Journal of Medical Ethics* 5 (1979): 141–42.

———. "Moral and Ethical Dilemmas in the Special Care Nursery." *New England Journal of Medicine* 289 (1973): 890–94.

Dworkin, Ronald. *Taking Rights Seriously.* Cambridge: Harvard University Press, 1977.

Dyck, Arthur. "An Alternative to the Ethic of Euthanasia," in R. M. Williams, ed. *To Live and To Die: When, Why, and How.* New York: Springer Verlag, 1973, 98–112.

Easton, David. *A Systems View of Political Life.* Chicago: University of Chicago Press, 1965, rev. ed. 1979.

———. *The Political System.* 2nd ed. Chicago: University of Chicago Press, 1981.

Easton, J. A. *Contributions to Legal Medicine: Being Observations on the Jurisprudence of Infanticide.* Edinburgh: Sutherland and Fox, 1852.

Ebenstein, William, et. al. *American Democracy.* New York: Harper and Row, 1967.

Englehardt, H. Tristram. "Aiding the Death of Young Children," in Marvin Kohl, ed. *Beneficient Euthanasia.* Buffalo: Prometheus Books, 1973, 180–92.

_____. "Defining Death: A Problem for Law and Medicine." *Annals of Respiratory Diseases* 112 (1975): 587–91.

_____. "Euthanasia and Children: The Injury of Continued Existence." *Journal of Pediatrics* 83 (1973): 7071.

_____. "Medicine and the Concept of a Person," in T. Beauchamp, ed. *Ethical Issues in Death and Dying.* Englewood Cliffs: Prentice, 1978.

Englehardt, Tristram, and Baruch Brody, eds. *Mental Illness: Law and Public Policy.* Boston: D. Reidel, 1980.

Ennis, Bruce, and Richard Emery. *The Rights of Mental Patients.* New York: Avon Books, 1978.

Feldstein, Paul. *Health Care Economics.* New York: John Wiley, 1982.

Finnie, John. *Natural Law and Natural Rights.* Oxford: Clarendon Press, 1981.

Fletcher, George. "Prolonging Life." *Washington Law Review* 42 (1967): 999–1016.

Fletcher, John. "Abortion, Euthanasia and Care of Defective Newborns." *The New England Journal of Medicine* 292 (1975): 75–78.

Foot, Philippa. "The Problem of Abortion and the Doctrine of the Double Effect." *Oxford Review* 5 (1967): 5–15.

Forkosch, Morris. "Privacy, Human Dignity and Euthanasia: Are These Independent Constitutional Rights?" *University of San Fernando Valley Law Review* 3 (1974): 1–25.

Fortescue, John. *The Governance of England: Otherwise Called the Difference between an Absolute and a Limited Monarchy.* Westport, Conn.: Hyperion Press, 1979.

Fost, Norman. "Counseling Families Who Have a Child with a Severe Congenital Anomaly." *Pediatrics* 67 (1981): 321–24.

_____. "Putting Hospitals on Notice." *Hastings Center Reports* 12 (August 1982): 5–8.

Frankel, M. *Criminal Sentencing.* New York: Hill and Wang, 1975.

Frankena, William. *Ethics.* Englewood Cliffs: Prentice Hall, 1964.

Freemen, John. "Is There a Right to Die—Quickly?" *Journal of Pediatrics* 80 (1972): 904–8.

Frisch, Morton, and Richard Stevens, eds. *American Political Thought.* New York: Scribners, 1970.

Fuller, Lon. *The Morality of Law.* New Haven: Yale University Press, 1968.

Gildin, Hilail. *Rousseau's Social Contract.* Chicago: University of Chicago Press, 1983.

Ginzberg, Eli. "The Social Security System." *Scientific American* 246 (January 1982), 51–57.

Glenn, Gary. "Abortion and Inalienable Rights in Classical Liberalism." *American Journal of Jurisprudence* 20 (1975): 62–80.

_____. "Hobbes on Inalienable Rights," paper given at the International Hobbes Tercentenary Conference, Boulder, Colorado, August 1979.

_____. "Inalienable Rights and Locke's Argument for Limited Government: Political Implications of a Right to Suicide." *Journal of Politics* 46 (1984): 81–105.

_____. "Inalienable Rights and Positive Government in the Modern World." *Journal of Politics* 41 (1979): 1056–80.

Glover, Jonathan. *Causing Death and Saving Lives.* London: Penguin, 1977.

Godwin, William. *Enquiry Concerning Political Justice.* Edited by K. C. Carter. Oxford: Clarendon Press, 1971.

Goldwin, Robert, ed. *A Nation of States: Essays on the American Federal System.* Chicago: Rand McNally, 1974.

Goodhart, C. B. "Estimation of Illegal Abortions." *Journal of Biosocial Science* 1 (1969): 235–45.

_____. "The Frequency of Illegal Abortion." *Eugenics Review* 55 (1964): 197–200.

Greenburg, David. "Involuntary Psychiatric Commitments to Prevent Suicide." *New York University Law Review* 49 (1974): 227–69.

Grisez, Germain. "Suicide and Euthanasia," in Horan and Mall, eds. *Death, Dying and Euthanasia*, 742–814.

Grisèz, Germain, and Joseph Boyle. *Life and Death with Liberty and Justice*. South Bend: University of Notre Dame Press, 1979.

Gutman, Amy. *Democratic Equality*. New York: Oxford University Press, 1979.

Haksar, Vinit. *Equality, Liberty and Perfectionism*. "Clarendon Library of Logic and Philosophy." Oxford: Oxford University Press, 1979.

Hanke, Lewis. *All Mankind is One*. De Kalb, Ill.: Northern Illinois University Press, 1974.

Hart, H. L. A. *The Concept of Law*. Oxford: Clarendon Press, 1961.

Hart, H. L. A., and A. M. Honoré. *Causation and the Law*. Oxford: Clarendon Press, 1958.

Hart, John Ely. *Democracy and Distrust*. Cambridge: Harvard University Press, 1980.

Hauerwas, Stanley. *Truthfulness and Tragedy*. South Bend: Notre Dame University Press, 1977.

_____. *Vision and Virtue*. South Bend: Notre Dame University Press, 1974.

Heffernan, Bart, M.D. "The Early Biography of Everyman." in Thomas Hilgers and Dennis Horan, eds. *Abortion and Social Justice*. New York: Sheed and Ward, 1972, 3–25.

Heiden, James, et al. "Severe Head Injury and Outcome," in A. J. Popp, ed., *Neural Trauma*. New York: Raven Press, 1979, 327–40.

Helmholtz, R. H. "Infanticide in the Province of Canterbury in the Fifteenth Century." *History of Childhood Quarterly* 1 (1974): 379–90.

Herberg, Will. *Protestant, Catholic, Jew*. New York: Doubleday, 1960.

Heymann, Philip, and Douglas Barzelay. "The Forest and the Trees: *Roe* v. *Wade* and Its Critics." *Boston University Law Review* 63 (1973): 765–69.

Heymann, Philip, and Sarah Holtz. "The Severely Defective Newborn: The Dilemma and the Decision Process."*Public Policy* 23 (1975): 381–417.

Hilgers, Thomas, and Dennis Horan, eds. *Abortion and Social Justice.* New York: Sheed and Ward, 1972.

Hilgers, Thomas, Dennis Horan, and David Mall, eds. *New Perspectives on Human Abortion.* Fredricksburg, Md.: University Publications of America, 1981.

Hinton, John. *Dying.* London: Penguin Books, 1972.

Hobbes, Thomas. *Leviathan.* Edited by M. Oakeshott. London: Collier Books, 1962.

Hobbins, J. C., et al. "Stage II Ultrasound Examination for the Diagnosis of Fetal Abnormalities with an Elevated Amniotic Fluid A-Fetoprotein Concentration," *American Journal of Obstetrics and Gynecology* 142 (1982): 1026–29.

Holdsworth, William. *A History of English Law.* London: Methuen, 1924.

Horan, Dennis, and David Mall, eds. *Death, Dying and Euthanasia.* Fredricksburg, Md.: University Publications of America, 1977.

Horan, Dennis, and M. Delahoyde, eds. *Infanticide and the Handicapped Newborn.* Provo, Utah: Brigham Young University Press, 1982.

Horwitz, Robert, ed., *The Moral Foundations of the American Republic.* Charlottesville: University of Virginia Press, 1977.

Hume, David. *Essays: Moral, Political and Literary.* London: Oxford University Press, 1963.

"In the Matter of the Treatment and Care of Infant Doe: Declaratory Judgment." *Connecticut Medicine* 47 (1983): 409–10.

Irani, K. D., and G. E. Meyers, eds. *Emotion: Philosophical Studies.* New York: Haven Publishing, 1983.

Jaffa, Harry. *Crisis of the House Divided.* New York: Doubleday, 1959.

———. *Equality and Liberty.* New York: Oxford University Press, 1963.

_____. *How to Think About the American Revolution*. Durham, N.C.: Carolina Academic Press, 1977.

Jaffa, Harry, and R. W. Johanson. *In the Name of the People*. Columbus: Ohio State University Press, 1959.

Jaffe, Frederick. "Enacting Religious Beliefs in a Pluralistic Society." *Hastings Center Report* 8 (August 1978): 15.

Jarvis, Judith Thompson. "A Defense of Abortion." *Philosophy and Public Affairs* 1 (1971): 47–66.

Jay, John, Alexander Hamilton, and James Madison. *The Federalist*. New York: Modern Library, 1941.

Jefferson, Thomas. *Notes on the State of Virginia*. Edited by William Peden. Chapel Hill: University of North Carolina Press, 1955.

Jenkins, I. *Social Order and the Limits of Law*. Princeton: Princeton University Press, 1980.

Johanson, R. W., editor. *The Lincoln–Douglas Debates*. New York: Oxford University Press, 1965.

Johns, N. "Family Reactions to the Birth of a Child with a Congenital Anomaly." *Medical Journal of Australia* 5 (1971): 277–81.

Jones, Gary. "Rights and Desires." *Ethics* 92 (1981): 52–56.

Jonson, Albert, and Michael Garland, eds. *Ethics of Newborn Intensive Care*. Berkeley: Institute of Governmental Studies, University of California, 1976.

Jonson, Albert, and Michael Garland. "A Moral Policy for Life/Death Decisions in the Intensive Care Nursery," in Jonson and Garland, *Ethics of Newborn Intensive Care*, 142–55.

Jordan, Winthrop. *White over Black*. Chapel Hill: University of North Carolina Press, 1968.

Kamisar, Yale. "Some Non-Religious Views Against Proposed Mercy Killing Legislation." *Minnesota Law Review* 42 (1958): 969–1042.

Kant, Immanuel. *Political Texts*. Edited by H. Reiss. Cambridge: Cambridge University Press, 1970.

"Karen Ann Quinlan: A Family's Fate." *Washington Post*, 26 May 1981, 1.

Kellum, Barbara. "Infanticide in England in the Later Middle Ages." *History of Childhood Quarterly* 1 (1974): 367–78.

Kendall, Wilmore. "The Open Society and Its Fallacies." *American Political Science Review* 54 (1960): 972–79.

Kennedy, Edward. "Toward a New System of Criminal Sentencing: Law with Order." *American Criminal Law Review* 16 (1979): 353–83.

Kenney, A. "Intention and Purpose in Law," in R. Summers, ed. *Essays in Legal Philosophy.* London: Oxford University Press, 1968, 146–63.

Kluge, E. W. *The Ethics of Deliberate Death.* Port Washington, N.Y.: Kennikat Press, 1981.

Kobler, A. "Suicide: Right and Reason." *Bioethics Quarterly* 2 (1980): 46–55.

Kohl, Marvin. *The Morality of Killing.* New York: Humanities Press, 1974.

_____. "Voluntary Death and Meaningless Existence," in Kohl, ed. *Infanticide and the Value of Life.* Buffalo: Prometheus Books, 1979, 210–11.

_____., ed. *Beneficient Euthanasia.* Buffalo: Prometheus Books, 1975.

_____., ed. *Infanticide and the Value of Life.* Buffalo: Prometheus Books, 1979.

Kolata, G. B. "Mass Screening for Neural Tube Defects." *Hastings Center Report* 10 (December 1980): 8–10.

Koppleman, L., and J. Moskop, eds. *Ethics and Mental Retardation.* Boston: D. Reidel, 1984.

Koppleman, L. "Respect and the Retarded," in L. Koppleman and J. Moskop, eds. *Ethics and Mental Retardation.* Boston: D. Reidel, 1984, 65–85.

Korein, Julius. "The Problem of Brain Death." *Annals of the New York Academy of Science* 315 (1978): 19–38.

Kraepelin, E. *Manic Depressive Illness and Paranoia.* Edinburgh: E. and S. Livingstone, 1924.

Kuflik, A. "The Inalienability of Autonomy." *Philosophy and Public Affairs.* 13 (1984): 270–98.

Ladd, John, ed. *Ethical Issues Relating to Life and Death.* New York: Oxford University Press, 1979.

Langer, William. "Checks on Population Growth: 1750–1850," *Scientific American* 226 (February 1982): 92–99.

Laslett, P., and W. G. Runciman, eds. *Philosophy, Politics and Society.* 2nd Series. London: Barnes and Noble, 1961.

Lebacqz, Karen. "Prenatal Diagnosis and Selective Abortion." *Linacre Quarterly* 40 (1973): 109–27.

Lester, D. "Attempts to Predict Suicidal Risk Using Psychological Tests." *Psychiatry Bulletin* 74 (1970): 1–17.

_____. "The Relationship of Mental Disorder to Suicidal Behavior." *New York State Journal of Medicine* 71 (1971): 1503–5.

Lewis, A. "Melancholia: A Clinical Survey of Depressed States." *Journal of Medical Science* 80 (1934): 277–378.

Litman, Robert. "Beyond Crisis," in Edwin Schneidman, ed. *Suicidology: Contemporary Developments.* New York: Grune and Stratton, 1976.

Litman, Robert, Norman Faberow and Edwin Schneidman. *The Psychology of Suicide.* New York: Science House, 1970.

Locke, John. *An Essay Concerning Human Understanding.* Edited by P. Nidditch. Oxford: Clarendon Press, 1976.

_____. *Letter on Toleration.* Edited by Charles Sherman. New York: Appleton-Century Crofts, 1937.

_____. *Two Treatises of Government.* Edited by Peter Laslett. Cambridge: Cambridge University Press, 1960.

Lorber, J. "Results of Treatment of Myeolomeningocele." *Developmental Medicine and Child Neurology* 13 (1971): 279–303.

Macintyre, Alastair. *After Virtue.* South Bend: Notre Dame, 1979.

Mall, David, and Dennis Moran, eds. *Death, Dying and Euthanasia.* Baltimore: University Publications, 1975.

Mannes, Marya. *Last Rights.* New York: Signet, 1975.

Mansfield, Harvey. "Thomas Jefferson," in Morton Frisch and Richard Stevens, eds. *American Political Thought.* New York: Scribners, 1970.

Matson, Donald. "Surgical Treatment of Myelomeningocele." *Pediatrics* 42 (1968): 225.

McClone, David, and James Brown. "Treatment Choices for the Infant with Meningomyelocele," in D. Horan and M. Delahoyde, eds. *Infanticide and the Handicapped Newborn.* Provo, Utah: Brigham Young University Press, 1982, 69–75.

McCormick, Richard. "A Proposal for Quality of Life Criteria for Sustaining Life." *Hospital Progress* 59 (1975): 76–79.

_____. "Notes on Moral Theology." *Theological Studies* 44 (1983): 119–22.

_____. "To Save or Let Die." *Journal of the American Medical Association* 229 (1974): 172–76.

McGuire, Daniel. *Death by Choice.* New York: Schocken Books, 1973.

McLone, D. G., M.D. "Press Release," *Americans United for Life*, 5 December 1983.

Menzel, Paul. "Are Killing and Letting Die Morally Different in Medical Contexts?" *Journal of Medicine and Philosophy* 4 (1979): 269–93.

Montesquieu, Baron de. *Persian Letters.* Translated by J. R. Loy. New York: Random House, 1962.

_____. *Spirit of the Laws.* Translated by T. Nugent. New York: Hafner Publishing Co., 1949.

Morris, Arval. "Law, Morality and Euthanasia for the Severely Defective Newborn," in M. Kohl, ed. *Infanticide and the Value of Life.* Buffalo: Prometheus Books, 1979, 137–58.

_____. "Voluntary Euthanasia." *Washington Law Review* 45 (1970): 239–71.

Murphy, G. "Clinical Identification of Suicide Risk." *Archives of General Psychiatry* 27 (1972): 356–60.

New York Times, September 18, 20, 22, 30, October 21, 30, November 2–4, 8, December 6–9, 1983; January 8, 1984.

Noonan, John. *A Private Choice.* New York: Free Press, 1979.

_____., ed. *The Morality of Abortion.* Cambridge: Harvard University Press, 1970.

O'Rourke, K. "Lessons from the Infant Doe Case." *Connecticut Medicine* 47 (1983): 411–12.

Paris, John. "Terminating Treatment for Newborns: A Theological Perspective." *Law Medicine and Health Care* 12 (1982): 120–24.

Patterson, Edwin. *Jurisprudence.* Brooklyn: Foundation Press, 1953.

Pearlman, Robert, et al. "Variability in Physician Bioethical Decisionmaking: A Case Study of Euthanasia." *Annals of Internal Medicine* 97 (1982): 420–25.

Peel, John, Malcolm Potts, and Peter Diggory. *Abortion.* New York: Cambridge University Press, 1977.

Perkins, R. *Criminal Law.* St. Paul: West's Publishing Co., 1968.

Perlin, S., ed. *Handbook for the Study of Suicide.* London: Oxford University Press, 1975.

Perry, Michael. "Abortion, Public Morals and the Police Power: The Ethical Function of Substantive Due Process." *UCLA Law Review* 23 (1976): 689–736.

Peterson, Peter. "The Coming Crash of Social Security." *New York Review of Books* 29 (4 December 1982): 34–39.

_____. "The Salvation of Social Security." *New York Review of Books* 29 (December 16, 1982): 50–57.

Petrie, A. *Individuality in Pain and Suffering.* Chicago: University of Chicago Press, 1967.

Pincoffs, Edmund. "Quandary Ethics." *Mind* 80 (1971): 552–71.

Pitkin, Hanna. *The Concept of Representation.* Berkeley: University of California Press, 1972.

Plato. *Apology.* Translated by H. Tredennick. Baltimore: Penguin Books, 1954.

_____. *The Laws.* Translated by Thomas Pangle. New York: Basic Books, 1979.

_____. *The Republic.* Translated by Allan Bloom. New York: Basic Books, 1968.

_____. *The Statesman.* Translated by J. B. Skemp. Indianapolis: Bobbs-Merrill, 1957.

Popkin, Richard. *The History of Skepticism from Erasmus to Spinoza.* Berkeley: University of California Press, 1979.

Popper, Karl. *The Open Society and Its Enemies.* rev. ed. 2 vols. London: Oxford University Press, 1961.

Pound, Roscoe. "Justice According to Law." *Columbia Law Review* 13 (1913): 706.

The President's Commission for the Study of Ethical Problems in Medicine and Biomedical and Behavioral Research.

Deciding to Forego Life Sustaining Treatment. Washington, D.C.: US Government Printing Office, 1983.

———. *Defining Death*. Washington, D.C.: US Government Printing Office, 1981.

Rachels, James. "Active and Passive Euthanasia." *New England Journal of Medicine* 292 (1975): 78–80.

———. "Euthanasia," in T. Regan, ed. *Matters of Life and Death*. New York: Random House, 1980.

Ramsey, Paul. "The Case of the Curious Exception." In Paul Ramsey and Gene Outka, eds. *Norm and Context in Christian Ethics*. New York: Charles Scribners, 1967, 67–135.

———. *Ethics at the Edges of Life*. New York: Columbia University Press, 1978.

———. *Patient as Person*. New Haven: Yale University Press, 1970.

Rawls, John. *A Theory of Justice*. Cambridge: Harvard University Press, 1971.

Regan, Donald. "Rewriting *Roe* v. *Wade*." *The Law and Politics* of Abortion. Edited by M. Vinoviskis and C. Schneider. Lexington: D. C. Heath, 1980.

Regan, T., ed. *Matters of Life and Death*. New York: Random House, 1980.

Reich, Warren. "Quality of Life and Defective Newborn Children," in Chester Swinyard, ed. *Decision Making and the Defective Newborn*. Springfield: Charles Thomas, 1978, 489–511.

Reiser, Stanley. "The Dilemma of Euthanasia in Modern Medical History," in Bok and Behenke, eds. *Dilemmas of Euthanasia*, 29–49.

Robertson, John. "Involuntary Euthanasia of Defective Newborns." *Stanford Law Review* 27 (1975): 213–69.

Robinson, N., and H. Robinson. *The Mentally Retarded Child*. New York: McGraw Hill, 1976.

Rosen, A. "Detection of Suicidal Patients: An Example of Some Limitations on the Prediction of Infrequent Events." *Journal of Consulting Psychology* 18 (1954): 397–403.

318

Rosen, G. "History," in S. Perlin, ed. *Handbook for the Study of Suicide.* London: Oxford University Press, 1975, 3–29.

Rousseau, Jean-Jacques. *Emile.* Edited by Alan Bloom. New York: Basic Books, 1980.

_____. *The Government of Poland.* Translated by F. Watkins. New York: Nelson, 1953.

_____. *Letter to D'Alembert.* Translated by Alan Bloom. Glencoe, Ill.: Free Press, 1960.

_____. *The Social Contract.* Translated by L. Blair. New York: Mentor Books, 1974.

Russel, O. R. *Freedom to Die.* New York: Human Sciences Press, 1975.

Ryn, Claes. *Democracy and the Ethical Life.* Baton Rouge: Louisiana State University Press, 1976.

Sartorius, Rolf. "Paternalistic Grounds for Involuntary Civil Commitment: A Utilitarian Perspective." In Tristram Englehardt and Baruch Brody, eds. *Mental Illness: Law and Public Policy.* Boston: D. Reidel, 1980., 137–45.

Schneidman, Edwin, ed. *Suicidology: Contemporary Developments.* New York: Grune and Stratton, 1976.

Schulz, R. "Effects of Control and Predictability on the Physical and Psychological Well Being of the Aged." *Journal of Personality and Social Psychology* 33 (1976): 563–73.

Shapiro, S. R. "Medical Treatment of Defective Newborns." *Harvard Journal on Legislation* 20 (1983): 137–52.

Shaw, A., et al. "Ethical Issues in Pediatric Surgery: A National Survey." *Pediatrics* 60 (1977): 588–92.

Shaw, Anthony. "Dilemmas of Informed Consent in Children." *New England Journal of Medicine* 289 (1973): 885–89.

Sherlock, Richard. "Competency and Social Rationality." *Journal of Medicine and Philosophy.*

_____. "For Everything there is a Season: The Right to Die in American Law." *Brigham Young Law Review* No. 2 (1982): 545–616.

_____. "The Right to Die as Public Policy: A Review." *Political Science Reviewer* 10 (1982): 251–86.

Singer, Marcus. *Generalization in Ethics*. New York: Alfred Knopf, 1961.

Singer, Peter. "President Reagan and Baby Doe." *New York Review of Books*. 9 March 1984.

Skeel, Joy, and Ron Benson. "Medical Indications for Postponing Death," paper delivered at meeting of the American Academy of Religion, at New Orleans, La., 1978.

Slater, Eliot. "Choosing the Time to Die," in M. F. Battin and D. Mayo, eds. *Suicide: The Philosophical Issues*. New York: Macmillan, 1980, 200–206.

Smith, G. K., and E. D. Smith. "Selection for Treatment in Spina Bifida Cystica." *British Medical Journal* 4 (1973): 189–93.

Spinoza, Baruch. *Ethics*. Translated by R. H. Elwes. New York: Dover Books, 1951.

———. *The Political Treatise*. Translated by R. H. Elwes. New York: Dover Books, 1951.

Sprott, S. E. *The English Debate on Suicide: From Donne to Hume*. Lasalle: Open Court, 1961.

Social Security in America's Future: The Final Report of the National Commission on Social Security. Washington, D.C.: US Government Printing Office, 1982.

"Statement of the AMA to DHHS: Handicapped Infants." *Connecticut Medicine* 47 (1983): 417–20.

Steele, W., and J. Hill. "A Plea for the Legal Right to Die." *Oklahoma Law Review* 29 (1976): 328–48.

Steinbock, Bonnie. "Baby Jane Doe in the Courts." *Hastings Center Report* 14 (February 1984): 13–19.

———., ed. *Killing and Letting Die*. Englewood Cliffs: Prentice Hall, 1979.

Stevas, Norman St. John. *Life, Death and the Law*. Bloomington: Indiana University Press, 1961.

Storing, Herbert. "Slavery and the Constitution," in Robert Horwitz, ed., *The Moral Foundations of the American Republic*. Charlottesville: University of Virginia Press, 1977.

Strauss, Leo. *Liberalism: Ancient and Modern*. New York: Free Press, 1963.

_____. *Natural Right and History.* Chicago: University of Chicago Press, 1953.

_____. *On Tyranny.* Ithaca: Cornell University Press, 1963.

_____. *The City and Man.* Chicago: Rand MacNally, 1964.

Stravino, V. D. "The Nature of Pain." *Archives of Physical Medicine* 51 (1970): 37–44.

Strong, Carson. "Defective Infants and Their Impact on Families: Ethical and Legal Considerations." *Law Medicine and Health Care* 13 (1983): 10–15.

_____. "Positive Killing and the Permanently Unconscious Patient." *Bioethics Quarterly* 3 (1981): 190–205.

Suckiel, Ellen. "Death and Benefit in the Permanently Unconscious Patient." *Journal of Medicine and Philosophy* 3 (1978): 38–52.

Swinyard, Chester, ed. *Decision Making and the Defective Newborn.* Springfield: Charles Thomas, 1978.

Syska, Barbara, Thomas Hilgers, and Dennis O'Hare, "An Objective Model for Estimating Criminal Abortions and Implications for Public Policy," in Thomas Hilgers, Dennis Horan, and David Mall, eds. *New Perspectives on Human Abortion.* Fredricksburg, Md.: University Publications of America, 1981, 164–81.

Szaz, Thomas. "The Ethics of Suicide."*Antioch Review* 3 (Spring 1971): 7–17.

Taub, S. "Medical Decisionmaking for Defective Infants." *Connecticut Medicine* 47 (1983): 413–16.

Thomas, C., and W. A. Fitch. "The Exercise of Discretionary Decisionmaking by the Police." *North Dakota Law Review* 54 (1977): 61–98.

Tooley, Michael. "A Defense of Abortion and Infanticide," in Joel Weinberg, ed. *The Problem of Abortion.* Belmont, California: Wadsworth Press, 1973, 51–91.

_____. "An Irrelevant Consideration: Killing versus Letting Die," in B. Steinbock, ed. *Killing and Letting Die.* Englewood Cliffs: Prentice Hall, 1979, 56–63.

_____. *Abortion and Infanticide.* New York: Oxford University, 1984.

Trammel, Richard. "Saving Life and Taking Life." *Journal of Philosophy* 72 (1975): 131–37.

_____. "The Presumption against Taking Life." *Journal of Medicine and Philosophy* 3 (1978): 53–67.

"Treating the Defective Newborn: A Survey of Physicians' Attitudes." *Hastings Center Reports* 6 (1976): 2–5.

Triche, Charles, and Diane Triche. *The Euthanasia Controversy 1812–1974: A Bibliography.* Troy, N.Y.: Whiston Publications, 1975.

Tribe, Laurence. *American Constitutional Law.* Mineola, N.Y.: Foundation Press, 1978.

_____. "Forward to the Supreme Court—1972 Term: Toward a Model of Roles in the Due Process of Life and Law." *Harvard Law Review* 87 (1973): 20–23.

Trowell, Hugh. *The Unfinished Debate on Euthanasia.* London: SCM Press, 1973.

Trubo, Richard. *Act of Mercy.* Los Angeles: Nash, 1973.

Tuck, R. *Natural Rights: Their Origin and Development.* New York: Cambridge University Press, 1979.

Ungar, Roberto. *Knowledge and Politics.* New York: Free Press, 1975.

_____. *Law in Modern Society.* New York: Free Press, 1975.

Veatch, Robert. "The Whole Brain Oriented Concept of Death: An Outmoded Philosophical Formulation." *Journal of Thanatology* 3 (1975): 13–30.

_____. *Death, Dying and the Biological Revolution.* New Haven: Yale University Press, 1976.

Walton, D. *On Death and Dying.* Montreal: McGill–Queens University Press, 1979.

Weber, Leonard. *Who Shall Live.* New York: Paulist Press, 1976.

Weinberg, Joel, ed. *The Problem of Abortion.* Belmont, California: Wadsworth, 1973.

Weir, R. F. "The Government and Selective Non-Treatment of Handicapped Infants." *New England Journal of Medicine* 309 (1983): 661–63.

_____. *Selective Non-treatment of Handicapped Newborns.* New York: Oxford University Press, 1984.

Werner, Oscar. *The Unmarried Mother in German Literature.* New York: Columbia University Press, 1917.

Werner, Richard. "Abortion: The Moral Status of the Unborn." Social Theory and Practice 3 (1974): 201–22.

Weschler, Herbert, and Jerome Michael. "A Rationale for the Law of Homicide," *Columbia Law Review,* 37 (1937): 701–53.

Williams, B. "The Idea of Equality," in P. Laslett and W. G. Runciman, eds. *Philosophy, Politics and Society,* 2nd Series. London: Barnes and Noble, 1962.

Williams, Glanville. *The Sanctity of Life and the Criminal Law.* New York: Alfred Knopf, 1957.

Williams, R. M., ed. *To Live and To Die: When Why and How.* New York: Springer Verlag, 1973.

Wilson, James. *Works.* Edited by Robert McClosky. Cambridge: Harvard University Press, 1967.

Windstrup, George. "Locke on Suicide." *Political Theory* 8 (1980): 169–82.

Wright, B. *Physical Disability: A Psychological Approach.* New York: Harper and Row, 1960.

Zuk, G. H. "The Religious Factor and Role of Guilt in Parental Acceptance of the Retarded Child. *American Journal of Mental Deficiencies* 64 (1959): 145–53.

Index

Authors

A.M.A. Council of Scientific Affairs 300 n37
Aaron, H. J. 281 n50
Ackerman, T. 279 n19
Al-Farabi 269 n6, 270 n13
Alvarez, A. 289 n2
AMA 282 n58
Amundsen, D. 283 n7
Anderson, J. G. 270 n10
Angell, M. 281 n57
Annas, G. 268 nn17-18, 288 n71
Applebaum, P. 291 n17
Aquinas, T. 269 n6
Aristotle 26-31, 225, 275 n36, 296 nn30, 32
Arras, J. 101, 280 n35, 281 n52, 282 n59
Ashley, B. 281 n42, 281 n46, 285 n34, 287 n56

Bagely, C. 291 n20
Bakan, D. 280 n28
Bannion, A. 281 n47
Barraclough, R. 178, 291 n14
Barrus, R. 270 n14
Barry, R. 289 n83
Barzelay, D. 293 n4
Battin, M. P. 293 n41
Beauchamp, T. 131, 285 n35, 290 n4
Becker, L. 205-6, 294 nn9-10, 294 nn11-12
Behenke, J. 282 n1
Behlmer, G. 277 n3
Benson, R. 287 n52
Bernat, J. 286 n46
Bersath, C. L. 281 n57
Beskow, J. 291 n15
Bickel, A. 293 n1
Blackstone, Sir W. 296 n31
Blackstone, W. 64, 274 n24
Blum, W. 292 n25

325

Boeyink, D. 280 n28
Bok, S. 282 n1
Bonhoeffer, D. 302 n1
Boyle, J. 129, 276 n47, 285 nn21, 25-26, 28, 286 nn41, 46, 292 n32, 293 n42, 295 n29
Brandt, R. 80, 269 n4, 278 nn10-11, 290 n12
Brody, B. 294 n13
Brown, J. T. 267 n3, 297 n12, 301 n38
Burt, R. 285 n32
Byrn, R. 133, 285 nn36-37

Campbell, A. G. 241, 277 n7, 280 n39, 297 n13, 298 n14
Cahill, L. 299 n28
Camus, A. 73, 289 n1
Cantor, N. 285 n34, 289 n88
Casey, L. 301 n39
Cassel, E. 98, 280 n30, 286 n43
Chambers, M. 267 n1
Childress, J. 254, 286 n42, 289 n82, 300 nn29-30
Cicero 269 n6, 270 n13
Cohen, R. M. 291 n17
Coke, J. 275 n40
Connecticut Medicine 281 n47, 282 n58
Connery, J. 281 n 57
Crane, D. 237-40, 287 n52, 297 nn4-10
Crenvik, A. 301 n40
Crocker, L. 289 n2
Cropsey, J. 270 n12, 296 n30
Crystal, S. 269 n8
Culver, C. 286 nn42, 46
Curran, W. 283 n9

Damme, C. 76, 277 n4
D'Arcy, E. 278 n15
D'Arcy, Eric 298 n20

De Grazia, S. 264, 302 n2
Delgado, R. 287 n55
Delhoyde, M. 277 n7
Destro, R. 296 n31
Devine, P. 274 n30
DHHS 109, 281 n49, 282 nn60-61
Diggory, P. 294 n14
Donne, J. 290 n4
Donnelly, J. 283 n9
Douglas, J. 70, 276 n49, 290 n10
Downing, A. B. 282 n1
Duff, R. 241-42, 277 n7, 278 n14, 280 n39, 285 n27, 297 n13, 298 nn14-15
Dworkin, R. 254, 299 n25, 300 n29
Dyck, A. 285 n39

Easton, J. A. 271 n19, 277 n5
Ebenstein, W. 296 n34
Ely, J. H. 293 n1
Emery, R. 178, 291 nn13, 18
Englehardt, H. T. 80, 186, 188-90, 278 n9, 292 nn32-33, 35-36, 293 n38, 286 nn44-45, 47, 287 n49
Ennis, B. 178, 291 nn13, 18

Faberow, N. 290 n3
Farber, B, 279 n17
Feinberg, J. 302 n42
Feldstein, P. 270 n10
Finnie, J. 299 n28
Fitch, W. A. 276 n45
Fletcher, G. 134, 285 n38
Fletcher, John 277 n7
Fletcher, Joseph 100, 280 n32
Flew, A. 186, 292 n33
Foot, P. 285 n27
Forkosch, M. 287 n55
Fortescue, J. 275 n40
Fost, N. 278 n15, 281 n52
Francis, L. 292 nn34, 37
Frankel, M. 276 n44

Cases

Subjects